PRAISE FOR *RAW FOOD FOR REAL PEOPLE*

"Rod's down-to-earth approach and his ability to simpli~~~~~~~~~~~~~~~~e out-standing. Raw food is healthy and delicious, and a~~~~~~~~~~~tes in *Raw Food for Real People*, it's for everyone."

— **BRENDAN BRAZIER,** pro~~~~~~~onman triathlete and author of *Thri~~ ~he Vegan Nutrition Guide*

"In his new cookbook, Rotondi is a welcome guide to eating raw and being real. He offers vibrant food alternatives for classic dishes, such as coleslaw and potato salad.... Rotondi's creative recipes can be thrown together by even the busiest chefs.... His easy sense of humor demystifies the process of arranging meals of living vegan foods."

— *LA YOGA*

"I've been enjoying Rod's delicious raw foods for years. It's a true win-win — good for my health and good for the environment. Rod has inspired me to adapt a good portion of my diet to raw."

— **ANDY LIPKIS,** founder of TreePeople

"Rod's food philosophy provides a guide to conscious eating for real people.... Rod is revealing the next evolution in raw food, and the possibilities are limitless. I invite you to enter a delectable adventure in raw dining."

— from the foreword by **MICHAEL BERNARD BECKWITH,** author of *Spiritual Liberation*

"The time has come for us to love ourselves enough to take action to heal ourselves. This book gives us the skills to do so."

— **RABBI GABRIEL COUSENS, MD, MD(H),** Diplomat of the American Board of Holistic Medicine, and Director of the Tree of Life Rejuvenation Center

"The solution to our country's health problems is simple and well within reach: eating a raw, alkaline, electron-rich diet as outlined in this book can ensure a consistently healthy, fit body free from *all* sickness and so-called disease, or dis-ease."

— **ROBERT O. YOUNG, PhD,** coauthor of *The pH Miracle*

RAW FOOD FOR REAL PEOPLE

RAW FOOD FOR REAL PEOPLE

Living Vegan Food Made Simple

ROD ROTONDI
Foreword by Michael Bernard Beckwith

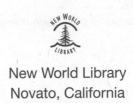

New World Library
Novato, California

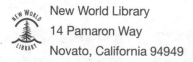 New World Library
14 Pamaron Way
Novato, California 94949

Text design by Mary Ann Casler
Typography by Tona Pearce Myers

Library of Congress Cataloging-in-Publication Data
Rotondi, Rod.
Raw food for real people : living vegan food made simple / by Rod Rotondi ; foreword by Michael
Bernard Beckwith.
     p.   cm.
Includes index.
ISBN 978-1-57731-974-0 (paperback : alk. paper)
1. Raw food diet. 2. Vegetarianism. I. Title.
RM237.5.R685 2009
613.2'6—dc22   2009027733

First paperback printing, November 2010
ISBN 978-1-57731-974-0
Printed in Canada on 100% postconsumer-waste recycled paper (exclusive of photo insert)

New World Library is a proud member of the Green Press Initiative.

10   9   8   7   6   5   4   3   2   1

To all the people who have suffered or are suffering from health challenges due to the food they eat. The good news is that the human body has an amazing ability, even after years of neglect and maltreatment, to rebound and renew itself when properly fed.

True wisdom consists in not departing from nature
and in molding our conduct according to her laws and model.
— **Lucius Annaeus Seneca**

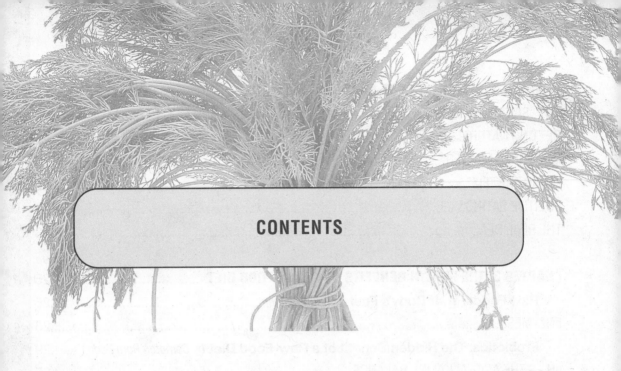

CONTENTS

Acknowledgments..xvii
Foreword by Michael Bernard Beckwith...xix

INTRODUCTION...1
ORGANIC FOOD..3
A VEGAN DIET..3
OUR RELATIONSHIP WITH FOOD..4
NOTES ABOUT THE RECIPES...7

CHAPTER 1. ROD'S RAW ROAD...9
LA FAMIGLIA...10
FRENCH HIGHS...12
FOREIGN INTRIGUES...13
THE RAW THAT BROKE THE CAMEL'S BACK...14
A TASTE FOR THE STATES...16
CALIFORNIA DREAMIN'..17

CHAPTER 2. HISTORY'S BEST-KEPT SECRET..19

THE "SAD" DIET..20

GETTING NATURAL...21

MIND OVER MATTER..21

FIXING THE "FIX"..22

POSITIVE EATING..22

THE REAL DEAL...23

CHAPTER 3. THE HEALTH BENEFITS OF A RAW-FOOD DIET................................25

   Raw Foods: Your Body's Fuel *by Brian Clement*................................26

ENZYMES..28

   Probiotics: The Hidden Benefit of a Raw-Food Diet *by Compton Rom Bada*.........29

pH — THE ACID-ALKALINE BALANCE...30

   A Raw Alkaline Diet: The Diet for Immortality and Freedom from

   All Sickness and Disease *by Robert O. Young*..............................31

OXYGEN...33

WATER..33

ANTIOXIDANTS...33

FIBER..33

ELECTROMAGNETIC ENERGY...34

   Preventing and Healing Diabetes with a Raw-Food Diet

      by Rabbi Gabriel Cousens..35

CHAPTER 4. TRANSITIONING TOWARD A RAW-FOOD DIET..39

DEALING WITH FOOD ADDICTIONS...40

DETOXING AND FASTING...42

CHAPTER 5. SETTING UP YOUR RAW-FOOD KITCHEN..45

BASIC EQUIPMENT..45

GOOD TO HAVE...46

STOCKING YOUR PANTRY...46

BE PREPARED...48
HELPFUL HINTS FOR PREPARING RAW FOODS.....................................49

CHAPTER 6. SPROUTING BASICS...53
GETTING STARTED...54
A WORD ABOUT NUTS..56
SPROUTING CHART..57

CHAPTER 7. DEHYDRATION: CRACKERS, CROQUETTES, PIZZA, AND BREAD.............61
CRACKERS..63
    Flaxseed Crackers..64
    Sicilian Savory Snaps..65
CROQUETTES..66
    Flying Falafel Croquettes...66
    Veggie Sun Burger Croquettes...67
PIZZA...69
    Pizza Pizzazz..69
    Pizza Pizzazz Abbondanza...72
    Italian Croutons...72
    Italian Herb Bread..72
BREADS..73
    Mango Bread...73
    Artisan Herb Bread...74

CHAPTER 8. GETTING STARTED: BREAKFAST...................................77
SMOOTHIES..77
    Nut Mylk..78
    Coconut Mylk..79
    Smoothie Recipes..81
PORRIDGES: OATMEAL AND BUCKWHEAT..83
    Real Deal Oatmeal...83
    Emerald City Oatmeal...84

Count Choco Maca Oatmeal..84

Living Buckwheat Porridge...84

Fruity Oatmeal or Buckwheat Porridge..84

Buckwheat Breakfast Feast..85

GRANOLA...86

Groovy Granola..86

Very Berry Granola..86

Tropical Granola...87

Choco Granola...87

CHAPTER 9. APPETIZERS..89

Nori Rolls with Atlantis Pâté...89

Miso Dulse Dip..91

Heirloom Tomatoes with Coconut Mozzarawla..................................92

Cashew Kreme Cheeze..93

Onion and Chive Cashew Kreme Cheeze..94

Kreme Cheeze and Lox...94

Mango and Coconut Cashew Kreme Cheeze......................................94

Cashew Kreme Cheeze Sliders..94

Baba Ganoush..95

Onion Rings..96

Rawvioli with Mushroom Sauce..97

CHAPTER 10. MAKING A SALAD A MEAL..99

Sprouted Chickpea Hummus...100

Sprouted Chickpea Hummus with Sun-Dried Tomatoes...................101

Sprouted Chickpea Hummus with Black Olives and Chives.............101

Holy Moly Guacamole..104

Hale Kale Salad..105

Caesar in the Raw Salad..107

Caesar in the Raw Wrap...108

Wakame Wonder Salad..109

Raw Slaw...109

Potatoless Salad with Lemon Dill Sauce...110

Wild Rice Pilaf...112

DRESSINGS...113

Leaf Organics House Dressing...113

Gluten-Free House Dressing..114

Really Raw Ranch Dressing...115

Pomegranate Dressing...116

A NOTE ABOUT OILS...117

WRAPS..117

Bedouin Burrito...118

CHAPTER 11. SOUPS...121

Middle Eastern Lentil Soup...122

Mexican Corn Chowder...123

Kids' Corn Chowder...123

Kreme of Butternut Squash Soup..124

Kreme of Asparagus Soup..125

Kreme of Mushroom Soup..126

Spanish Gazpacho...127

CHAPTER 12. ENTRÉES..129

Rawsagna..129

Rawsagna with Extras...131

Cannelloni...131

Pad Thai...132

Fishless Sticks...134

Raw Veggie Shish Kebab..136

Mediterranean Burgers with Pesto Sauce..137

Flying Falafel Sandwich with Coco-Curry Sauce..................................139

THANKSGIVING FEAST..141

Love Loaf...141

Cranberry Sauce..142

Mashed Taters...143

CHAPTER 13. DESSERTS...145

Lemon Zinger Cookies...145

Brownie Balls or Bars..146

Rocky Road Bananas...147

Strawberry Ice Kreme..148

Raspberry Vanilla Cheezecake..149

Raspberry Cacao Cheezecake...150

Cushy Carrot Cake...151

Really Raw Apple Pie...153

Strawberry Mousse Tartlets...155

Chocolate Brownie Sundae..156

Coco Cacao Maca Mousse..158

Coconut Macaroon Balls..159

CHAPTER 14. RAW FOOD FOR REAL KIDS WITH JEANNETTE ROTONDI......................161

IS RAW ENOUGH?...162

GROWING OUR KIDS...162

RAW BABY...163

TODDLER EATS...165

THE WELL-NOURISHED CHILD..166

Afterword: Food Is Family..169

Metric and Celsius Equivalents...171

Index..173

About the Author..185

Color photographs follow page 60.

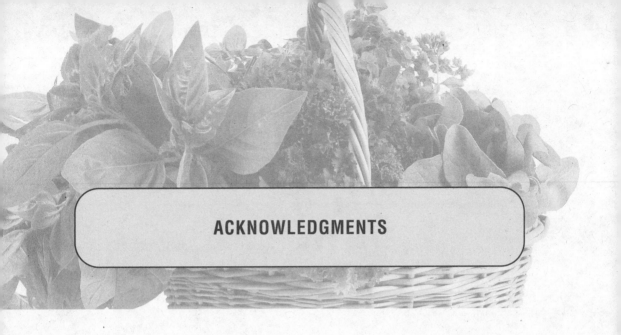

ACKNOWLEDGMENTS

First off, I wish to thank Marc Allen from New World Library for his support and the incredible company he has built. I greatly appreciate Georgia Hughes and Kristen Cashman, my fantastic editors, who went way beyond the call of duty in bringing this book to fruition.

I wish to thank my whole family for their love and support, but especially my dad, Roger Rotondi, for his unwavering support and for sharing his love of food and family. What a great heart!

I thank Jeannette Rotondi for being an amazing mother to our daughter, Lilli, and for her help with some of the scientific background for this book. And Lilli, thank you for joining us on this journey, putting it all in perspective, filling my heart with love, and making me laugh.

I also want to thank all my colleagues at Leaf Organics, especially Ray Gonzales, who has completely owned our mission to "Make it easy for people to eat healthy food."

It truly takes a village.

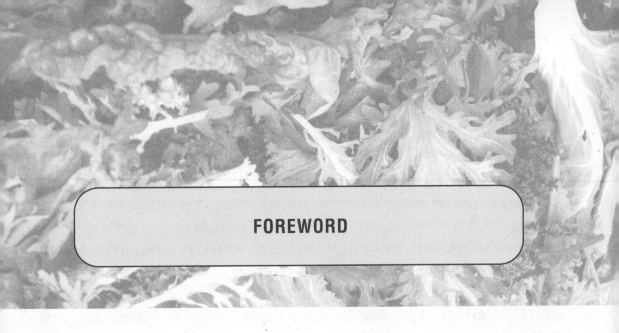

FOREWORD

Raw Food for Real People **delivers on its promise.** It offers a way of nourishing our-selves that delivers vibrant health and vitality. It also takes into account the emotional comfort we derive from food that satisfies both body and spirit. Rod's food philoso-phy provides a guide to conscious eating for real people.

People routinely comment on how healthy and energetic I am. One of the things I attribute my well-being to is that I prepare many of Rod's recipes at home — the recipes that are most frequently requested in his restaurants: amazing salads, savory sauces, smoothies, nourishing soups, desserts, dressings, and more. Rod's food aes-thetic, as well as his ethics and concern about how the Earth's resources are inextri-cably intertwined with how we grow, prepare, and eat our food, reminds us that eating is a sacred act, an art, and a spiritual practice of inner joy and satisfaction.

Ever since I began going to Rod's restaurant, Leaf Cuisine, four years ago, I have known I could trust him not only with my taste buds, but also with feeding me in a conscionable way. His preparations are in accord with my belief in placing sunlight-fed, organic foods into the body temple while respecting the environment by keep-ing it free of pesticides and synthetic fertilizers. The vision Rod presents of quality, purity, and enjoyment of our food is inspired by his commitment to the benefits of the raw-food lifestyle. My family and I have benefited so much from Rod's knowledge and love of foods that I extended an invitation to him to set up an outdoor food booth each Sunday at the Agape International Spiritual Center, the community I founded in Los Angeles in 1986. Upon experiencing Rod's cuisine, many individuals have changed the foods they eat and tell us regularly how their health, vitality, and well-being have greatly improved.

Today people are realizing that there are new choices to be made about food, as evidenced by the increased popularity of farmers' markets and the range of organic foods now available in traditional grocery stores. America's unhealthy relationship with food is evidenced by its expanding waistline as well as its increased incidence of childhood diabetes and other health issues. Today more than 50 percent of Americans admit to having been on a diet at one time or another. Increasingly we realize: *food choices matter*. Rod's holistic and fun approach to food education and preparation convinces us how optimal health can be realized through food choices rather than diets.

Eating a diet of raw food isn't a religion, and the raw-food style of living is not fanaticism. (In fact, Rod, I occasionally eat a juicy veggie burger — soy free of course — and it doesn't negate the benefits of my mostly raw diet.) The main point here is how Rod appreciates the beauty and pleasure of healthily prepared food and the messages — both subtle and overt — behind it.

As you turn the pages of *Raw Food for Real People*, you will see that his recipes are not complicated or time-consuming, and they use ingredients that can be found everywhere. While some foods may be new to you, most will be familiar ingredients that are being combined to give maximum nutritional value. Rod's recipes take food preparation from merely being time-consuming to being creative and offering maximum taste. Who doesn't appreciate the aroma of fresh herbs and the experience of heavenly food that is pleasing to the senses? Rod is revealing the next evolution in raw food, and the possibilities are limitless. I invite you to enter a delectable adventure in raw dining. You'll see how your whole personhood will shine with a new glow of radiant health — inside and out.

— **Michael Bernard Beckwith,**
author of *Spiritual Liberation: Fulfilling Your Soul's Potential*

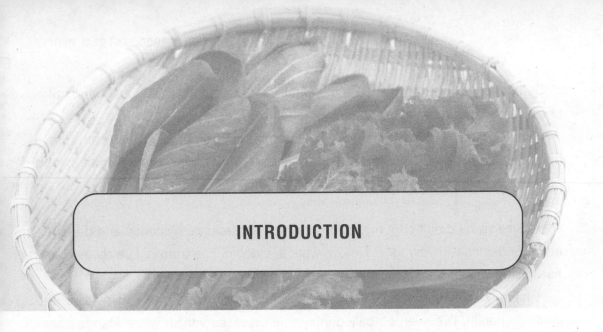

INTRODUCTION

Okay, I have three confessions to make up front.

CONFESSION ONE: First off, I have to admit that being a raw-food chef is easy. No, really. It's like *Dumb and Dumber* easy. I have experience with cuisines from around the world, and I can tell you that raw-food cuisine is the easiest ever.

The truth is that if you can cut an apple in half, you are a raw-food chef. And if you can slice or cube that apple, you qualify as a gourmet raw-food chef. So congratulations, chef, you have already graduated!

Oh, sorry — I'm supposed to say something here about the sacred and esoteric nature of raw-food preparation. About how we raw-food chefs meditate at least twelve hours per day and exercise by walking miles over flaming coals or large bodies of water.

But the truth is that most of what we do when preparing raw food is simple. In fact, it's best when it is simple. Let the food speak for itself. Plus, it's even easier to digest when it's simple. One could even argue that the whole idea of the raw-food movement is getting back to a simple and natural diet. Avoid adding too many cups of ego to your recipes. Simple dishes can still be incredibly elegant, delicious, nutritious, and artful.

What I am going to show you in this book is how to simply, deliciously, and nutritiously incorporate raw-food preparation into your life.

No, you don't have to take notes. Remember, it's simple. Our ancestors have been preparing food this way for millions of years — since long before blenders, food processors, and juicers entered our kitchens.

CONFESSION TWO: I didn't cure myself of a myriad of diseases, ailments, and degenerative conditions with raw food. I know, what a letdown. The truth is, I've always been healthy. I'm just much healthier and more vital when I eat raw food.

I have, however, witnessed firsthand the power of raw food to restore and enhance health. I've seen so-called incurable diseases vanish when friends abandoned cooked and highly processed foods in favor of healthier raw meals — including Leaf Organics foods. I can tell you I feel pretty good about that.

CONFESSION THREE: Since I discovered raw-food cuisine in 1996, I haven't always eaten a 100 percent raw-food diet. Sure, I did spend many of those years eating a purely raw-food diet, but there have been times when I chose to eat other foods as well. Perhaps it was emotional eating, or just enjoying different foods and cuisines. Perhaps it was to join in social situations. But whatever the reason, the point is, it's okay.

Adopting a raw-food diet is not about judging others or ourselves. It's not about good or bad. It's about things that work for us and things that don't. I have found consistently over the years that the more raw foods I eat, the better I feel and look — and I'm still pretty attached to feeling and looking good!

Conversely, I have found that the more cooked foods I eat, the worse I feel and look. It's that simple. There is a consequence to everything we do, and the consequences of poor eating can manifest themselves quickly.

My last name is Rotondi, which means "the round ones" in Italian. If I still ate the standard American diet, I know I would be grossly overweight and struggling with health challenges such as diabetes, which runs in my family. So while I didn't cure myself of any major illnesses, I attribute my good health and relatively youthful appearance to a diet predominantly made up of raw foods.

Next, I'll address two fundamental food choices that I believe are an integral part of the raw-food diet and lifestyle.

ORGANIC FOOD

As I see it, we have a choice. We can choose foods that have been treated with herbicides, pesticides, and fungicides and that may include genetically modified organisms (GMOs) and who knows what other kinds of chemicals, preservatives, and stabilizers; I call this slow suicide. Or we can choose unadulterated real foods from nature. To me, the choice of organic foods is integral to conscious eating and raw-food cuisine. A raw-food lifestyle is about eating pure food from nature and giving ourselves the best food possible. While the cost for organic products is a little higher, I view it as money I won't have to spend on visits to my doctor.

When we choose organic foods, not only are we keeping our own internal environment clean, but we also are being mindful of the global environment. Look at the extra money you spend on organics as a kind of tax to protect the future of our planet, because right now we are seriously polluting the land, water, and air with conventional agricultural practices. Every bite counts, both for our bodies and for the planetary body.

I feel so strongly about this that I would rather eat organic cooked foods than conventional raw foods. I just don't want to support the chemical agriculture system or put those chemicals in my body.

A VEGAN DIET

While there are raw foodists who include raw meats and dairy in their diets, the vast majority are vegans. If you haven't heard, there is a lot of new data pointing to the incredible health benefits of a vegan diet. Check out *The China Study* by Dr. T. Colin Campbell. It's a book about possibly the most comprehensive study of human nutrition ever undertaken, which concluded that, in Dr. Campbell's words, "People who ate the most animal-based foods got the most chronic disease. . . . People who ate the most plant-based foods were the healthiest and tended to avoid chronic disease. These results could not be ignored."*

---

* See the book's website, http://www.thechinastudy.com/about.html (accessed June 4, 2009).

According to the American Diabetes Association, vegetarian diets are associated with a reduced risk for obesity, coronary artery disease, hypertension, diabetes mellitus, colorectal cancer, lung cancer, and kidney disease. Additionally, virtually every health organization in existence advocates eating more fresh fruits and vegetables.

Then there is the idea of not killing other sentient beings in order to eat. It's a nice feeling to finish a delicious, nutritious, and satisfying meal knowing that no animal had to give its life for it — not to mention the fact that the vast majority of animals raised for consumption are born, bred, and killed in miserable conditions.

Or how about the fact that the livestock industry is one of the biggest polluters of all and is right at the top of the list of industries that contribute to global warming? Did you know that the single most effective thing any individual can do to minimize their negative effect on global warming is to eat less or no meat?

Here are a few of my favorite quotes about this.

"Nothing will benefit human health and increase the chances for survival of life on Earth as much as the evolution to a vegetarian diet." — **Albert Einstein**

"The greatness of a nation and its moral process can be judged by the way its animals are treated." — **Mohandas Gandhi**

"Until he extends the circle of his compassion to all living things, man will not himself find peace." — **Albert Schweitzer**

OUR RELATIONSHIP WITH FOOD

Many of us in this culture have lost our relationship with food. The only relationship many kids growing up today have with food is going to a drive-through or popping a package into the microwave.

This is a relatively new phenomenon. During the first half of the twentieth century — only a couple of generations ago — household vegetable gardens were commonplace, and many families raised animals for meat or milk. My paternal grandfather fed his family of thirteen children largely out of the garden his family tended and with the animals they raised.

To them, food wasn't an abstraction or simply a means of satisfying hunger. It was something they had an intimate relationship with long before it hit the dining room table. And right up to his last days, my grandfather used to love walking down to the garden, picking some ripe peppers and tomatoes, grabbing some freshly laid eggs from the hen coop, and coming back to the kitchen to cook up a scrambled egg, pepper, and tomato sandwich with some thick Italian bread.

I remember doing this with him, and I understood the great pleasure he got from it. Then he would show me his biceps and make them jump for me, and he'd say if I wanted to be strong I should eat good food from the garden, too. I'm not exactly sure how the couple of beers he would enjoy with that sandwich figured in, but I did understand the joy he felt in his relationship with and love of the Earth and its bounty.

While we don't all have the land or the time to grow a large garden, there are ways we can grow more of our food ourselves at home. One of the things we have done at our home was to pull up some of our lawn to make room for more vegetable garden space. We now grow greens such as arugula and herbs such as basil and oregano instead of grass.

Herb gardens are pretty easy to grow just about anywhere — even a large pot or window box will do fine. You can grow them from seed or buy seedlings at most garden supply stores. It's really fun to be able to run out to the herb garden to cut a few leaves of basil or pull up some spring onions when making a recipe.

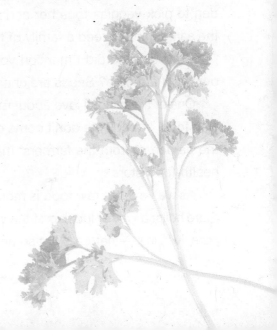

Sprouts are another really easy thing to grow. Later in the book I will teach you how to sprout legumes such as chickpeas and lentils as well as a host of seeds, nuts, and grains. One nice thing to try sprouting at home is sunflower seeds. They're super easy! Just put some seeds in some soil in your garden, pot, or window box, or even in an old wheatgrass tray, water them regularly, and in a matter of days you will have your own sunflower greens. These are ready when about 3 to 4 inches long, and they can be cut and added to a wrap or salad, or just eaten as is. They are very nutritious and can even be juiced.

One pot of sunflower seeds we were sprouting went unharvested for too long and we ended up with small sunflower plants. We transplanted them to the garden and are growing the whole plants, which are beautiful, and now we look forward to harvesting the seeds. What fun!

Of course, the other advantage of growing your own veggies, herbs, sprouts, and greens at home is the knowledge that your food is secure and nutritious. In this day and age, with scares about food security abounding, it's nice to know exactly what's been done to your food before it hits your plate.

My three-year-old daughter loves growing things. She is learning where food comes from and about the relationship between the Earth and ourselves. She loves to go out and pick some greens and then come back and lovingly make a salad with me or her mom. Who knows? One day she might take her grandchild out to the garden to pick veggies together and tell stories about her dad's grandfather, who did the same thing to feed a family of thirteen children during the Great Depression.

Oh yeah, and did I mention you can also save a lot of money by growing your own stuff at home? Seeds are cheap!

One of the things I love about raw-food cuisine is that it develops this relationship with food. Ingredients don't come out of a microwavable package; they come out of the garden or from the farmers' market or the organic produce section of the local health-food store.

As we've seen, raw food is more than just a cuisine — it's a lifestyle. It involves a more holistic way of looking at the world and our relationship to it. We see nature, and ourselves in it — nature is not something to be overcome but something to work with.

And once you start seeing food this way, it won't be long before you see everything this way.

NOTES ABOUT THE RECIPES

The recipes in chapters 7 through 13 of this book will get you on your way to becoming an accomplished raw-food chef. We cover all the bases — breakfast, appetizers, salads, soups, main courses, and desserts, plus the important raw-food practice of dehydration.

Please note that all the ingredients you use should be raw and preferably organic as well. Also, it's important to note that recipes for raw-food dishes tend to be more flexible than normal cooked-food recipes. This is because produce is almost always the main ingredient in raw-food recipes, and produce varies from season to season and region to region. Water content changes, as do size, taste, and so on. So to follow a recipe blindly really doesn't work. It's always important to consider all the variables and to adjust accordingly. If you are making a mousse and it's too runny, add more nuts. If you are making a dressing and it is too thick, add more liquid. Dehydration especially will vary depending on ingredients and environment. Things are going to dehydrate much faster on a dry, hot summer day than on a rainy, cold day. I suggest you use the recipes in this book as guides only — don't give up your own discernment and creativity.

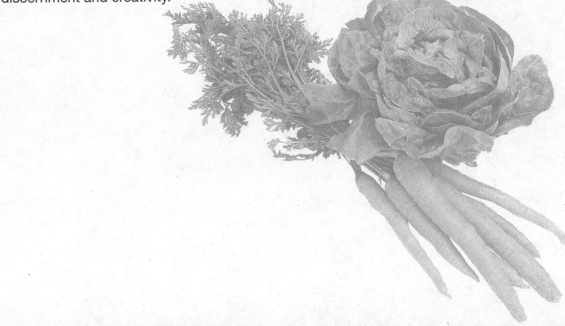

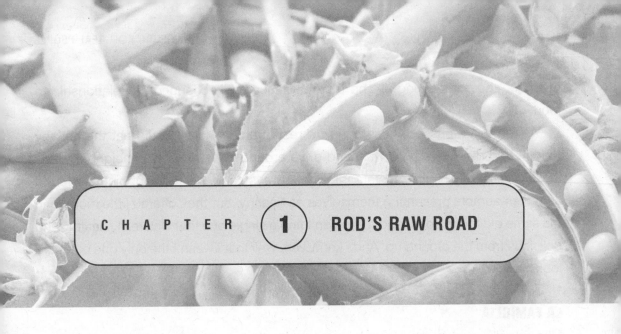

CHAPTER (1) ROD'S RAW ROAD

When I first discovered raw food in the 1990s, virtually no one had heard of a raw- or living-food diet. We were considered extremists, which I always found ironic considering we eat unadulterated, unprocessed foods from nature, whereas the standard American diet, what I call the "SAD" diet, is very far removed indeed from nature. Who's the extremist?

But all over the world, people are waking up to conscious eating, and the time to get back to real food is now.

I discovered raw and living foods in Greenwich Village in New York City in 1996. I was taking consciousness workshops back when the word *consciousness* wasn't used in every other sentence. The leaders of these workshops were eating raw food in order to "raise their vibrations," get clearer, and not be subject to food jags. I thought I would give it a try.

I soon found myself coming home with bags of beautiful fresh organic produce, seeds, nuts, and fruits I would use to prepare incredible meals and drinks. This led to a revelation. I was sitting down to one such meal — a dandelion-greens salad with pine nuts and pomegranate dressing — when it occurred to me that I was eating the food of the gods. I mean, when the gods get together for dinner, I don't think they do drive-through burgers. It is a cornucopia of vibrant, colorful, and life-filled fresh foods that I see the gods eating — and that realization really changed my relationship to food.

As the years passed, I searched for restaurants where I could eat the healthy foods I had discovered. I'd walk and drive around my surrounding neighborhoods looking for a truly healthy restaurant, but I always came back disappointed. I found some restaurants presenting themselves as healthy, but they offered little more than the same old thing repackaged. I couldn't find a single one that was really healthy and delicious from the ground up. And I knew very well that I wasn't the only one out there looking.

LA FAMIGLIA

Like virtually everyone out there, I have had family members and friends get sick and in some cases die from a myriad of degenerative diseases. On average, fifteen hundred Americans die every day from cancer. We have an epidemic level of obesity and diabetes in this country. And heart disease is accepted as a part of life. When I realized that food was the main culprit behind all this, I knew I was going to do something about it. I finally decided I would step into the breach and bring people what they were looking for — delicious, healthy food that is affordable and convenient.

I had a culinarily advantaged upbringing — I come from a predominantly Italian American family (with some Native American, Irish, and French thrown in). Food is central to our family culture. It's not only the reason we gather; it's also a passion. Everyone in my family cooks, not just the women. My father is an incredible baker, a genius with breads, pies, and pretty much anything else he puts his mind to. Some of my earliest childhood memories are of our family gathered together in the kitchen.

My dad used to enlist me, my sister, Joy, and my brothers, John and James, every holiday season to help him make pies. The oldest kids would help with peeling apples (competing for the longest apple-peel strip), and the younger kids would mix the sugar and spices

I learned important lessons about food from my dad. Because he is an engineer, he would break down the important factors in any recipe and explain (at length!) both the aesthetic considerations and the hard science behind his techniques and methods. I remember while I was working in Jerusalem for the UN, I asked my dad to send me his recipe for apple pie, because I wanted to get it exactly right. He wrote me back with a multipage treatise about apple pies. I can still make a beautiful classic apple pie, but one of my favorite culinary validations was when my dad tried my raw apple pie at Leaf and loved it.

I also was lucky enough to be exposed to other cuisines because of family connections. When I was ten years old, my mom arranged for my sister and me to spend a summer in Mexico with family friends. Then I spent my twelfth, thirteenth, and fourteenth summers in Rome, where my grandfather was the U.S. ambassador.

Because my family has a strong work ethic, we all had jobs, and mine was to help with food service. I was trained in formal food presentation and assisted with dinners, cocktail parties, and so on. And I became close with the head chef at the ambassador's villa, Dino, one of the best chefs in Italy. I used to hang out in the kitchen, learning about cooking and having fun with food and friends.

Of course, we used to eat pretty well those summers. The whole family would plan the menu for the next week. In the early mornings, I used to go to the local open-air markets with my grandmother, who was very hands-on in managing the embassy's hospitality. She always tried to get the best and freshest ingredients at the best prices. She was big on not wasting anything. In a way, I think she was a true conservationist. Today everyone is going green. Back in my grandmother's day, it was just considered common sense. One of her favorite sayings was "Waste not, want not." As I write, she is ninety-seven and still going strong.

Which leads me to introduce one of my favorite culinary skills — resourcefulness. My grandmother always said cooks are measured by what they can do with leftovers. The great ones can create delicious meals without a recipe, using the limited ingredients at hand. I always feel the resourcefulness challenge with raw foods, since this cuisine is in the process of being reinvented, or at least rediscovered, and the foods and ingredients one can use are limited compared to those in other cuisines. The resourcefulness and inventiveness required of a raw-food chef is partly why raw food appeals so strongly to me.

When my sister, Joy, and her then-husband were living on a sailboat in St. Thomas, Virgin Islands, she invited me, my girlfriend at the time, and my parents to join them for a week. We had a great time sailing around the islands. And we created a contest. Every day a different couple would make lunch and dinner. At the end of the week we voted for the best chef pair, and despite the tough competition, my team won. That's pretty serious validation. I think we won because of our resourcefulness and creativity.

The only time I had greater validation was when I entered a culinary contest in Marblehead, Massachusetts. Every summer they hold the Marblehead Culinary Arts Festival, a black-tie food competition among all the prestigious restaurants in the region. It's held outside in an old fort overlooking the harbor full of sailboats, and judged by five-star chefs from Boston's most celebrated restaurants. When they announced I had won both best of show and best theme, I was too shocked to say anything.

Another really great culinary validation came when I made homemade gnocchi for my nana (grandmother), and she said it was the best she had ever tasted. How good is that? We have a special family technique for making gnocchi, and it is still one of my favorite things to make for (and teach to) people I really like. Yes, I know, it's not raw, but it is part of my culture and family tradition, and people really love it!

My sister is arguably the most knowledgeable chef in the family. She knows everything about food. In fact, she used to own and run a business called Foodies.com, which offered lots of interesting information about food.

To give you an idea of the kind of culinary culture I grew up in: when my siblings and I were teenagers coming home from a late night and wanting a midnight snack, we would typically cook up a sauce from scratch and make pasta. No Hot Pockets for us!

FRENCH HIGHS

My culinary vistas matured greatly when I was sixteen and my family moved to Paris. Those teenage years in Paris were critical to my culinary education. The French love their food and take great pride in it. I was enthralled enough to sign up for French cooking courses at a local school. I learned how to make *pintade aux choux* (guinea fowl with cabbage) and a proper chocolate mousse, how to reduce a sauce, and much more.

My cousins, who happened to be living in Paris at the same time, love to tell the story of how I invited them over for a meal during a weekend that my parents were away. They said they were expecting peanut butter–and-jelly sandwiches but instead got a four-course gourmet French meal.

I loved all parts of the experience — even going to the local markets and bargaining for the best ingredients. Getting people I like together to share a meal is still one of my very favorite things to do.

Also, Paris is a very cosmopolitan city, with cuisines from all over the world. I received an amazing education in Algerian, Vietnamese, Chinese, Japanese, and other world cuisines. My siblings and I used to make weekend excursions to little hole-in-the-wall restaurants throughout the city. For a couple of bucks per person, one could find an incredible variety of great meals.

FOREIGN INTRIGUES

After returning to the States to go to college and then to graduate school, I volunteered for a year of grassroots development work with an American nonprofit agency. I spent a few months working all around Morocco, and then one year in Tunisia. Naturally I learned all about Moroccan tagines (clay-pot dishes) and about the differences between the two countries' couscous. I also learned all about beekeeping while managing projects teaching subsistence farmers how to use modern beekeeping methods. I had some incredible meals in the most rustic and pastoral of settings. I even completed the fasting month of Ramadan, breaking the day's fast every evening with friends and colleagues.

In Jerusalem, where I lived and worked for the United Nations Development Program (UNDP) for six years, I greatly enjoyed the Palestinian cuisine. With strong influences from Lebanon, Egypt, and the Bedouin culture, Palestinian cuisine is wonderfully delicious. I learned to make many dishes, held numerous dinner parties, and was invited to countless feasts in both the most sophisticated and simple environs.

It was in Jerusalem that I first became a vegetarian. My brother James came for a visit, and we took an eight-day trip to Egypt and back on my Honda XRV 650 African Twin motorcycle. Arabic cuisine includes wonderful vegetarian dishes, and we tried everything, including a sublime meal in a restaurant serving Nabatean food on the banks of the Nile in Aswan, where the Arab and African worlds meld.

At the UNDP, my job as program management officer was to help develop private business and agriculture in the West Bank and Gaza Strip. I worked with many food-related businesses, including a citrus-processing facility in Gaza; irrigation, bee-keeping, and cottage-industry food-processing projects; a chick hatchery; and the tourism industry. I was welcomed into homes and institutions without reserve. I still feel incredibly grateful for the hospitality I received and the insights I gained during this time of service.

It wasn't an easy job. Economic development work is never easy. And when it is done under military occupation and in the midst of an *intifadah* (a popular uprising), economic development is incredibly challenging. Under these trying circumstances, I saw some of the best and worse in human nature.

THE RAW THAT BROKE THE CAMEL'S BACK

Eventually I decided to experience firsthand the challenges and rewards of building a business in the third world. I had led the setup of the first business development center in the West Bank and Gaza Strip, trained many business consultants, and assisted numerous Palestinian businesses. But I had never owned my own business.

I had never experienced the challenge of making payroll or starting an enterprise from scratch, and I hadn't faced the specific hurdles entrepreneurs in economically and politically challenged areas must deal with. I decided to strike out on my own and "take a walk in the shoes" of the small businessmen and -women I had worked with as a UN program management officer. My business wouldn't be located in Gaza or the West Bank, however, but rather in a nearby area I had come to love.

I traded in my three-piece suit for a swimsuit and opened a scuba diving shop and resort in the Sinai. Yes, the Sinai — that wilderness where Moses wandered for forty years. Having been there and enjoyed the spectacular beauty of the Sinai, I imagined that Moses and the Israelites weren't really lost — they loved the area and were reluctant to leave!

Leaving Jerusalem, my home of six years, I loaded up my 1973 Land Rover Series 3 long bed, which I had rescued from the Samarian desert, with all my belongings and moved to a little Bedouin village called Dahab — Arabic for "gold" — nestled on a palm tree–lined bay on the Red Sea. Dahab had no paved roads, phones, or electricity when I arrived. It was a favorite stopover for backpackers and travelers, and I loved it. During the six years I worked for the UN in Jerusalem, I estimate I took at least fifty short trips to the Sinai — mostly to Dahab, where I practiced free diving and scuba diving.

The first thing I did after moving to Dahab was to take a scuba diving–instructor course. Next I partnered with an Austrian friend who was in the midst of establishing a diving center at a spectacular dive site. That's how the Canyon Dive Club was born — only the third diving center in Dahab, and the first to be owned by non-Egyptians. In the next years I went on to establish the Fantasea Dive Club, Club Red Divers, and Dive Zone.

We were the pioneers of Camel Diving Safaris, leading groups of tourists by camel up and down the Sinai coast to virgin dive sites. These were amazing trips that left indelible impressions on all who participated. Imagine riding up the coast on a camel with your own Bedouin guide with no signs of civilization — just rocky mountains to one side and the deep blue of the Red Sea to the other. We would camp overnight and make a fire and cook food for all. It was always a party, and the complete solitude brought immediacy to every breath. Plus the stars out there were absolutely stunning. With no man-made light for miles, the starlight was awe inspiring in its brilliance.

In the mornings we would be awakened by the Bedouin cooking bread over the fire and the sun rising over the mountains of Saudi Arabia on the other side of the Red Sea. After breakfast we would don our diving gear and venture into the water and a world of sparkling color and vibrant life. These were so much more than vacations — they were adventures into a world almost forgotten by modern man.

I spent about seven years in Dahab. It was an amazing time. When I look back now, it seems like another lifetime — one whose memory I treasure, but also one I find difficult to translate to my life in America. It was not only a different part of the world and a different culture and way of life; it's almost as if it was from a different time and space.

Our first dive center was only the third in Dahab, but by the time I left, in 2000, there were over fifty diving centers. "Progress" had arrived in force, and not in the way I had hoped and worked for.

Nevertheless, I spent some of the greatest years of my life in Dahab. And it was at one of my dive centers, Club Red, that I started my first restaurant, a little Italian place where my friend Enzo Ferraro was chef, making only fresh handmade Italian pasta. We later expanded to include a larger international menu — eventually even including raw food.

The full story of my experiences in the Middle East could be a book on its own, which I hope to write someday. My almost fifteen years there changed me forever. But at a certain point, I knew it was time for me to return home.

A TASTE FOR THE STATES

After a couple of weeks staying with friends in Copenhagen, I flew back to Boston and the warm embrace of my family.

The very next day I took a long walk around the town my parents were living in, Marblehead, Massachusetts. I happened upon a health-food store and went in to look around. It turned out they had a small restaurant area in the back that was vacant. When I say "small," I mean really small — room only for a tiny kitchen and a few tables. This was to be the spot for my first fully raw restaurant, Rod's Wrap and Juice Bar.

Before I launched Rod's, I worked as a manager/consultant for a raw-food restaurant in nearby Beverly, Massachusetts, called the Organic Garden. What I saw there clarified for me the importance of creating a clear identity in a restaurant. The Organic Garden was somewhere between a fancy sit-down restaurant and a café-style place. But it was neither one nor the other, and though it did serve some great food, the split personality was a problem. I decided to create a place with a clear identity, and I knew I wanted a place that was informal, quick, and affordable.

In fact, Rod's Wrap and Juice Bar was the first incarnation of what was to become Leaf Organics. It was there I created most of the recipes and the overall concept of a place focused on wraps, salads, smoothies, juices, and desserts — very simple but delicious food.

The town took to Rod's Wrap and Juice Bar immediately. Much to my surprise, my little place became a nexus of all the health- and spiritual-minded people of the area. This impressed upon me the importance of sharing food to the way we socialize. The "breaking of bread" is an age-old tradition, one that people often miss in our fast-paced culture.

Within months, I seemed to know everyone in town. I admit I did stand out a little at the time, with my shoulder-length dreadlocks. Before long, Rod's Wrap and Juice Bar was a going venture.

As I mentioned, every summer in Marblehead they hold a Culinary Arts Festival, in which all the best restaurants in the area compete. Despite the modest nature of my place, I decided to enter. Each establishment had a six-foot table upon which to present its offerings. A good friend helped me create a meadow scene with pallets of wheatgrass, flowers, and dishes of simple foods like guacamole, hummus, and fruit pies. I was honored simply to be part of the event, and when they announced I had won the two highest awards, it began to dawn on me that I was pretty good at this food thing.

CALIFORNIA DREAMIN'

While on the verge of opening Rod's Wrap and Juice Bars in other Boston-area neighborhoods, I took a trip out to California and realized this was the perfect place to plant the seeds of my quick-service raw-food concept. Southern California has perfect weather, lots of outdoorsy, athletic, and health-conscious people, and the best organic produce anywhere.

And sure enough, after completing a general-manager stint opening and running a raw-food restaurant in Santa Monica, I opened Leaf Cuisine on October 17, 2004, in Culver City, California, to lines stretching out the door. A year later, I opened our second location, on Ventura Boulevard in Sherman Oaks.

In my initial business plan, I had foreseen packaging our food and selling it to natural-food retailers. In the first years of running the restaurants, I had many requests from retailers to do this, but I held off. I wanted to focus on the restaurants until I felt totally ready to take on the packaged-food business.

Finally, in October 2006, I launched Real Live Foods Inc., which is licensed to produce and distribute Leaf Organics foods. We started with some wraps, salads, and dips and soon added desserts, dressings, crackers, and croutons. Initially we sold only to a few local stores, but we quickly expanded to Mother's Markets in Orange County, and then made it into California Whole Foods Markets.

Whole Foods has been a great partner in expanding our business, and it has proven to be the best means to get our optimally healthy food out to the most people in the quickest time. In fact, we just started a program to provide Leaf Organics burgers made to order at Whole Foods Market delis. We are in most of the Whole Foods Markets in California, Arizona, and Nevada (as well as many independent markets and other chains) and are in the process of expanding to the rest of the country.

In 2007, I began preparing everything for a Leaf Organics franchise offering, but I found that we had run out of production capacity due to the runaway success of our packaged-food line. So we established a state-of-the-art production facility in downtown Los Angeles, near the produce market. We distribute our products as far north as Sacramento and expect to hit most of the West Coast by the end of the year. We also intend to renew our restaurant chain expansion by opening more restaurants that we own and manage as well as through franchising.

Our intention is to bring both our packaged foods and our restaurants to every place that people want our style of optimally healthy food. And that area seems to be growing daily. This book and the DVD series we have also made available are part of our effort to show people how they can make this food and live this lifestyle for themselves. It's all about making it easy for people to eat the healthiest food possible.

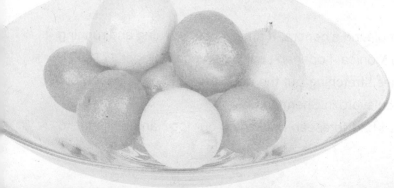

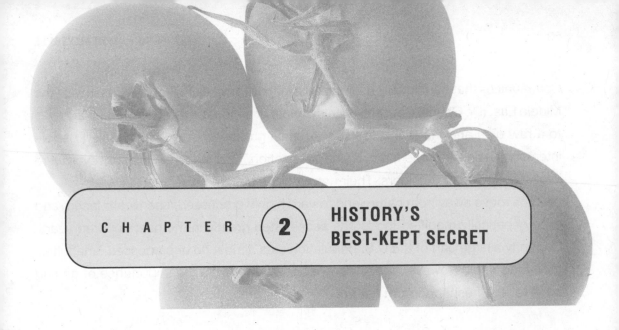

Some people think raw food is a new thing — a cutting-edge way of eating, newly discovered by scientists or Hollywood trainers for optimal beauty and health. In fact, a
raw diet is not new. It is not the latest craze. Hominids have evolved over seven million years, and for the vast majority of that time we ate only raw, living foods.

This original and longest-lasting human diet comprised primarily fruits, berries,
nuts, seeds, vegetables, and greens. It was all food from nature — unprocessed and
unadulterated. Meat was eaten only occasionally, primarily when scavenged or
during periods of drought when normal plant foods were unavailable. (There is con-
flicting evidence about the time period and frequency of early hominid meat consumption.) This is the way our ancestors ate until they discovered fire.

After the discovery of fire, humans began cooking their food as well as eating
meat more regularly (after all, uncooked meat is very hard to eat with human teeth).
The use of fire to process food before eating is a relatively new phenomenon in our
history.

Since the discovery of fire, we have strayed far from our original natural diet. But
the shift away from raw foods has been gradual and has varied among populations
based on their locations, natural resources, and cultures.

Some groups managed to buck the trend toward cooked and processed foods.

Communities that traditionally maintained a largely raw diet include the Essenes in the Middle East (Dr. Gabriel Cousens is an example of a modern-day Essene who adheres to a raw diet) and the Rishis in India — small groups of spiritually focused people interested in enlightenment and divine connection. Their experiences, however, were largely unknown to outsiders. Their natural diets became a secret.

The move away from nature and toward highly processed, chemically laced, and even genetically modified foods has accelerated greatly in the past hundred years. Currently a large part of the U.S. population eats almost no unprocessed, unadulterated food at all. However, today people are waking up to the importance of getting back to real, fresh food from nature.

THE "SAD" DIET

Today, as a matter of course, most of us eat foods that are far from their natural states. I call this the SAD, or standard American diet. We shop in convenience or grocery stores where the vast majority of food is highly processed. We fill our shopping carts with foods that have been heated to several hundred degrees, or mixed with additives whose names are impossible to pronounce. We stock our kitchens with foods that have been sitting on a shelf or in a warehouse for months and even years. We cheerfully buy foods that have been irradiated or pumped full of pesticides, herbicides, and fungicides, and in eating them we are committing a slow form of suicide.

In our world today, a person who eats exclusively foods still in their natural states might be considered an extremist. Think about that. It's considered completely healthy and normal to eat animal flesh pumped up with growth hormones and who knows what else. It is normal to eat food that has been packaged in plastic, bathed in chemicals, or irradiated in a microwave. Yet in our society, people who eat foods from nature are considered weird and a little threatening!

But that's changing. The secret is getting out.

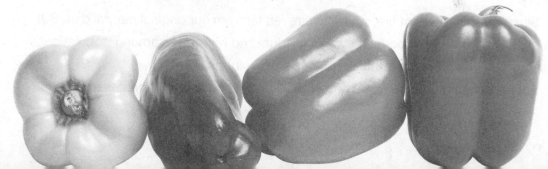

GETTING NATURAL

The raw-food diet is about getting natural — about rediscovering the natural way for humans to eat. Because despite all the knowledge of humankind — all our science and technology — what will make us healthiest and happiest is to eat the foods that nature, in its wisdom, has provided. Thinking we are smarter than nature is simply arrogant and, in fact, not very smart.

So what does it mean to eat from nature? It's not really that complicated. Actually, it's very simple. What is perhaps not so simple is to let go of many of the foods we are used to eating — and in fact often are addicted to eating, even when they don't really work for us.

Yes, we can become addicted to foods. Foods can affect our bodies as powerfully as drugs. And, like drugs, foods can create addictions.

So how do you know if a food is truly from nature? Let's try a simple test.

Hold a food item in your hand — for example, a powdered doughnut. Okay, while holding the powdered doughnut in your hand, ask yourself, Can I find this in nature?

I don't know about you, but I've never seen a doughnut tree or bush or plant. So a powdered doughnut is not from nature.

Now, hold an apple in your hand. . . .

Okay, I think you get it. This part is easy.

Now, after identifying your natural food, eat it. Eat the apple. It tastes good. No problem. Except (and this is the hard part) you are still hungry.

MIND OVER MATTER

After you eat your healthy apple, your mind might start telling you about all the things you are not getting. Things like protein, protein, and protein — this country is obsessed with protein! How many people do you know who have been rushed to the hospital with a protein deficiency? People are dying in droves every day from degenerative diseases brought on by the unnatural foods they eat — especially excessive meat. But what do we panic about? Protein deficiency!

So, here you are, thinking that maybe along with your apple you should eat some meat or cheese or eggs or something with lots of protein. Not because eating any of those things is on the whole very healthy. Not because your body needs them — it is possible to meet our modest protein needs with legumes, seeds, nuts, and plants. No, like most of us, you've simply been brainwashed from a very early age about the need to eat lots of protein from meat, eggs, and dairy.

What I am saying is that a big obstacle to eating naturally is the mind. When the mind gets out of the way, the body is remarkably good at determining what it needs to eat. Of course, before we can get to that level of body wisdom, we have to pass through the stage of kicking the food addictions virtually everyone has.

FIXING THE "FIX"

One of the most common food addictions is to refined sugar. Chances are good that you have been eating highly processed sugar products since you were a small child. Cookies, candy, soda, and sweets were probably given to you as treats, to reward good behavior or celebrate special occasions. It's no wonder, then, that as an adult you still feel you really need that sugar fix to make it through the day.

Intellectually you know you don't need it, but your body is telling you in very strong language that sugar is important to you. The good news is that, as with any addiction, if you can go without a fix for a period of time, the yearnings go away.

POSITIVE EATING

Now this is beginning to sound like a very uncomfortable process, right? You're beginning to think, Well, maybe this is not for me. So it's around this time, when you begin thinking that switching to a healthy raw-food diet might not be for you, that I like to remind people of one simple fact. And it's such an important fact that I am going to write it in bold.

Human beings are the only animals on Earth that cook their foods.

Think about that. Then think about this: human beings are the only animals who suffer from a high incidence of degenerative diseases and other health challenges such as cancer, heart disease, stroke, and diabetes.

There is a connection here! These facts are related!

Now I'm not saying we must eat every little item of food completely raw if we want optimal health. I'm not saying that eating raw is a panacea for modern humankind. However, I am saying that ultimately a primarily raw-food diet is our natural way to eat and, if done correctly, will bring us maximum health and happiness.

I add the caveat "if done correctly" because it is also possible to have a very unhealthy raw-food diet. It's like a guy who eats only Doritos and thinks he's eating healthy because he is ostensibly a vegetarian.

Vegetarianism may be defined by what you don't eat, and that can seem like deprivation. If you want to shift to a primarily raw diet and achieve optimal health, you need to start thinking of a raw diet in terms of what you do eat, as opposed to what you don't. You have an opportunity to focus on the amazing possibilities of a raw-food diet and can look forward to the wonderful benefits of feeling light, healthy, and energized.

THE REAL DEAL

All right, so what are the amazing possibilities? Like, how many ways can you prepare raw carrots and celery? I want to tell you that there is a whole cuisine that has been largely forgotten but is being rediscovered — and it is delicious! In raw cuisine, we can create virtually every taste and texture without adulterating the food.

Raw-food cuisine has rediscovered some of the oldest and healthiest food preparation techniques known to humankind, such as sprouting and low-temperature dehydration. Did you know that the way humans first made bread is the same way we make it at Leaf Organics?

First, people soaked their grains, then they rinsed them and let them sprout over a couple of days. Then they mashed them up, perhaps adding some salt or herbs for flavor. Then they would make them into cakes and put them on a rock in the sun. They'd go off and work in the fields or hunt, and at the end of the day, the bread would be "cooked." Just the action of the heat and air would dehydrate the food, leaving it crispy on the outside but warm and yummy on the inside.

In this kind of bread, the digestive enzymes are not killed. The food retains its natural nutrients — in fact, soaking and sprouting the grains greatly increases their nutritional benefits for the body.

In raw-food cuisine, we do the same thing. We make things like bread in a low-temperature dehydrator instead of on a rock, but it is the same process. The dehydrator simply blows warm air over a tray of food, slowly and simply removing much of the moisture. It's very slow. It might take eight to ten hours. But what's the rush?

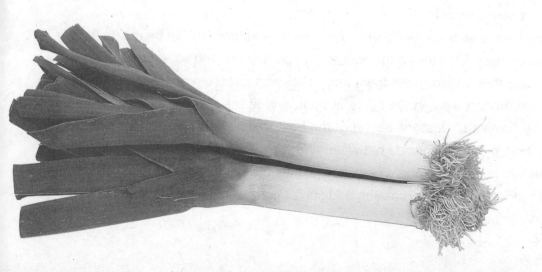

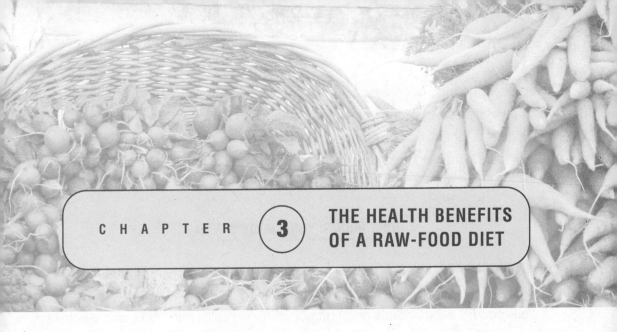

People today are incredibly confused about what to eat. We seem to have lost the thread of culture and tradition that used to inform our food choices. Every animal in nature knows exactly what to eat, yet modern humans, supposedly the smartest of animals, are confused and eat foods that are far from nature.

This book will not present a scientific treatise on why to eat raw foods. I am not a scientist (and I don't even play one on TV). However, I do believe in the wisdom of nature, and when it comes to food choices, I think the wisest course is to listen to our bodies first and foremost.

However, like most people interested in a raw-food diet, I ended up researching its nutritional aspects, to better understand the science behind the "aha" moment I had in 1996 when I decided to go raw. Being neither a scientist nor a nutritionist, I turned for information to the most trusted and experienced leaders in this field, including Dr. Gabriel Cousens of the Tree of Life Rejuvenation Center in Arizona, Dr. Brian Clement of the Hippocrates Health Institute in Florida, Compton Rom Bada of Ascended Health Products, and Dr. Robert O. Young, the author of *The pH Miracle* and other books. These highly trained doctors have spent decades using natural methods, and in particular a raw-food regime, to treat people with a myriad of ailments and often heal them. Their many books and articles have informed most of what I know about raw-food nutrition.

I present here an overview of some of the subjects related to this topic — in my words as well as those of the four experts mentioned above, who were kind enough to write sidebars for this book. I encourage you to read more of the work of these exceptional leaders in the field, to deepen your understanding of the science behind raw food.

RAW FOODS: YOUR BODY'S FUEL

BRIAN CLEMENT, PHD, LN, NMD, director of the Hippocrates Health Institute

Your body is a remarkable gathering of 95 trillion cells, microbes, and electrical charge. It perpetually renews itself as cells die and are born, and all of them mix with microbes from the environment in which you reside. Anatomy is constantly changing and evolving based on a number of influences. Organs, skeletal structure, blood chemistry, and microbes together create the human system. This system is not static but quite alive and requires ongoing nutritional input that addresses, develops, and grows the anatomy on several levels. Structurally, vitamins, minerals, proteins, and essential fatty acids all create the visible concrete matter that we see in totality as you. At a basic yet profound level, the functions of the system depend on hormones, oxygen, phytonutrients, and enzymes as their food and fuel, and in the case of phytonutrients, as their protectors. This banquet of elements is 100 percent available when the raw food that they are contained in has not been altered or processed.

Within raw, fresh, organic, plant-based fare lives a smorgasbord of nutritional elements that fully support the human anatomy. When you process, cook, or chemicalize your cuisine, you lose in total or at least in great part the appropriate nutrients that support the dynamic bioelectric system that houses your person. Correct nutrition not only offers the bland elements but also harbors the electric ionic frequencies appropriate to be ingested and utilized by your cells. This high frequency is completely neutered when food is heated above approximately 115°F (46°C). When your system receives electrically charged nutrition from raw foods, it both develops structural strength and impels each cell and organ to move forward in rhythmatic functioning. The energy from your ingested fare is what permits every part of your whole to maximize its abilities. For more than half a century, the institute that I have had the privilege to direct, Hippocrates Health Institute, has conducted research on hundreds of thousands of people as they adopted a raw-food diet. This often results in eliminating and preventing disease and certainly halts premature aging.

The twenty-first century is the time when our culture will renew its scientific understanding of food as medicine. *Orthomolecular* is a recently established term that describes the use of nutrients in conquering and preventing disease. If you want to live a healthy, long, fruitful, and happy life, one of the unwavering essential contributions is the commitment to consume uncooked plant-based food.

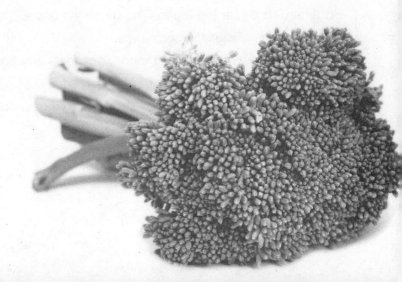

ENZYMES

Until fairly recently, most people had little understanding of the important role enzymes play in our bodies. But though they've often been overlooked, they are in fact the workhorses of our bodies. Enzymes are involved in virtually every metabolic process.

There are two major types of enzymes, metabolic and digestive. As author Edward Howell details in his book *Enzyme Nutrition*, we are born with a finite supply of enzymes in our body. When we use them, we are drawing from a finite "bank account" of enzymes.

The related scientific fact to understand is that every food comes with its own perfect complement of digestive enzymes. So, for example, if you cut an avocado in half and put it on the counter, it will start to break down because it has its own digestive enzymes within it. And because avocados also have a lot of wonderful plant fats, one of the enzymes they contain is lipase, which breaks down fat in the body. It's really quite an amazing system.

The thing is, these digestive enzymes are heat sensitive. The prevailing rule of thumb is that digestive enzymes die at around 118°F. Recent studies show some differences regarding the heat levels at which different digestive enzymes die, and that some may live to a significantly higher temperature. However, 118°F is the highest temperature we know for certain that digestive enzymes can survive.

What this means for us is that when we cook foods at elevated temperatures (above 118°F), we kill their digestive enzymes. As a result, our bodies have to work extra hard to digest the foods. The pancreas especially is stressed, having to make up for the loss of digestive enzymes.

After eating a meal of living foods, one feels energized and renewed. After eating a meal of cooked foods, one often feels tired and sluggish. Many believe that this is due to the body having to work extra hard to digest cooked foods.

PROBIOTICS: THE HIDDEN BENEFIT OF A RAW-FOOD DIET

COMPTON ROM BADA, founder of Ascended Health Products

(AscendedHealth.com)

Lately we have all heard a lot about probiotics, which literally means "for life." They are the beneficial microbes, or good bacteria, already present in our bodies — mostly in our guts but also in our mouths and skin — that help our bodies digest food, make vitamins, ward off diseases, and heal. We provide these bacteria with a good home, except when we take antibiotics (literally, "against life"), which clear out our guts — of the good bacteria as well as the bad.

Researchers now recognize these beneficial microbes as an essential part of the complex ecosystem we call the human body. In fact, we cannot live without them. Studies show that of the 100 trillion cells that make up the body, 90 percent are microbes. Unfortunately, evidence suggests that our body's probiotic microbe population naturally declines with age.

One way to counteract that tendency is to take probiotic supplements. Another is to eat raw foods. Everything we eat and drink contains lots and lots of bacteria, and live sprouts, leaves, fruits, and vegetables are the best sources of live, beneficial microbes. These good microbes are also found naturally in the soil — where plants grow. When we eat raw foods, we ingest some of the beneficial bacteria present in the soil. Traditional cooked food and fast food, on the other hand, contain bacteria that are harmful. Basically, cooking our food kills off the good bacteria. However, when we ingest only raw foods, our guts become so flooded with these good bacteria that the bad ones get "booted out." In some cases, deliberately consuming bacteria (in foods or supplements) can be more healthful than trying to kill off bacteria with antibiotics.

A recent landmark study, published in April 2008 in *Nature*, showed that people eating raw foods lead longer, healthier lives than those eating diets high in meat, processed foods, fat, and sugar. Indeed, diets high in raw foods have been shown to eliminate one form of diabetes and to vastly lower the incidence of cancer and heart disease. Other studies show that people with diabetes and heart disease who switched to a raw-food diet started to slowly reverse their symptoms, regardless of their genetic predisposition or ethnicity.

In short, the reason behind the epidemic of gut-borne illness in the United States is this: too many antibiotics and too much bad food create too much bad bacteria in our guts. We can change this dynamic by consistently ingesting beneficial bacteria to counteract the bad. (Note that eating cultured foods based on dairy, such as yogurt and cheese, will not help you in this regard.)

So put your health on the fast track by ingesting raw foods high in beneficial microbes. Start pushing out the bad bacteria and replacing them with the good!

pH — THE ACID-ALKALINE BALANCE

Another important health benefit of a raw-food diet is how it affects your body's pH — its acid-alkaline balance. Your body wants to be somewhat alkaline. It is more difficult for diseases to develop in an alkaline body. Also, many people feel better when alkaline; their aches and pains may be lessened or gone. Their mood is better. Their energy seems to flow more vigorously.

A well-balanced raw-food diet is predominantly alkaline, especially when green leafy vegetables play a significant role. This is one reason green juices are so wonderful.

You can actually buy pH test strips at the pharmacy and use them to test your body's pH with saliva or urine. Then try eating raw, with plenty of greens, for a couple of days, and check your pH again. It's amazing how well it works. But if you listen closely to your body, you won't need the pH strips to be able to notice the benefits.

By the way, one of the major food groups of the standard American diet, animal protein — be it red meat, poultry, or seafood — is acid producing! For more information on the relationship between raw foods and pH balance, see the sidebar by Dr. Robert Young on the facing page.

A RAW ALKALINE DIET: THE DIET FOR IMMORTALITY AND FREEDOM FROM ALL SICKNESS AND DISEASE

ROBERT O. YOUNG, PHD, coauthor of *The pH Miracle*

Of all the balances a healthy human body strives to maintain, the most crucial is the one between acid and base, or alkalinity. The body is meant to be alkaline, and it will go to great lengths to maintain the appropriate, slightly basic nature of its blood and tissues. But all body functions, including eating and drinking, produce acidic effects, so it is all too easy for blood and tissues to become acidic. That is, the human body is alkaline by design and acidic by function. The body is vulnerable to germs only when it is acidic — in a healthy alkaline environment, germs can't get a foothold. The idea is to keep the body alkaline by eliminating dietary and metabolic acids, thereby preventing the biological transformation of body cells into germs and ensuring radiant health.

The relationship between acid and base is scientifically quantified on a scale of 0 to 14 known as "pH," which stands for "potential hydrogen." On that scale, 7 is neutral. Below 7 is acid, and above it basic, or alkaline. Technically, pH reflects the concentration of hydrogen ions (positively charged molecules, protons, or acids) in any substance or solution. You don't need to understand all the details of the chemistry here. Just know that these two kinds of chemicals — acids and bases — are opposites, and when they meet in certain ratios, they cancel each other out, creating a neutral pH.

All foods and drinks have a pH value. Foods saturated with hydroxyl ions, or electrons, are alkaline. Foods saturated with hydrogen ions, or protons, are acidic. In this way, the pH scale is also a measurement of the electrical energy in food or drink. Cooked and processed foods, abundant in the standard American diet, are acidic, creating a huge dietary imbalance and a massive overacidification of cells, tissues, organs, and eventually, blood. This imbalance underlies all so-called disease, and general "dis-ease" as well. Eating a proper alkaline, electron-rich, raw diet and making healthy lifestyle choices are the only ways to prevent the imbalance. Eating raw alkaline foods also aids digestion and boosts your overall energy.

Fortunately for us, it is easy to categorize which foods are alkalizing. In general, animal foods (meat, eggs, and dairy), processed and refined foods, yeast products, fermented foods, sweet fruits, chocolate, and natural and artificial sugars are acidifying, as are alcohol, coffee, black tea, and sodas. Grains are acidifying, though a few (millet, buckwheat, and spelt) are only very mildly so. On the other hand, vegetables — especially green raw vegetables — and low-sugar fruits are alkalizing. Avocado, tomato, cucumber, and bell pepper are alkalizing as well. A few non-sweet citrus fruits, such as grapefruit, lemon, and lime, are also basic in the body, as are sprouted seeds, nuts, and grains.

The solution to our country's health problems is simple and well within reach: eating a raw, alkaline, electron-rich diet as outlined in this book can ensure a consistently healthy, fit body free from *all* sickness and so-called disease, or dis-ease. That is why I call this raw, alkaline diet the diet for immortality.

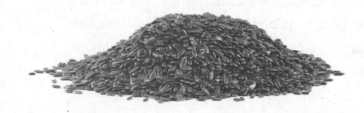

OXYGEN

The human body receives oxygen not only from the air we breathe but also through our skin and from our food. When we cook our food, we remove much of the oxygen stored in it. Getting enough oxygen into the body is a critical factor in good health.

WATER

While food is clearly critical to our health, we should also keep in mind that the human body is around 70 percent water. But despite having all kinds of new and better waters and water purifiers on the market, perhaps the best water in the world for humans is the water we get from plants. This water has been filtered by the plants. When we cook foods at high temperatures, we remove much of their water. Eating foods raw allows you to take in the natural water in the foods. In fact, when eating a raw-food diet, you may find you don't need to drink as much liquid, because you are getting a lot from your food. However, proper hydration is key to good health, so be sure to get enough liquids. One of my favorite ways to hydrate is by drinking young coconut water, which is also a natural source of electrolytes.

ANTIOXIDANTS

Metabolic processes involving oxygen can produce pollutants commonly known as *free radicals* that can damage our bodies. There are special nutrients known as *antioxidants* that seek out the free radicals and neutralize or destroy them, thus preventing or at least diminishing negative effects, and in some cases even reversing damage. Free-radical damage is often cited as a contributing factor in diabetes, cancer, macular degeneration, and heart disease. When we eat lots of fresh foods, we have a constant stream of antioxidants entering the body to help neutralize free radicals. And hey, here is some really good news — raw cacao (read: chocolate) is super high in antioxidants!

FIBER

One of the most important factors in good health is proper elimination. It's a bit awkward for people to talk about, but it is critical for feeling our best and creating a healthy internal environment. Wastes need to be removed from the body. Fortunately, our bodies are equipped with a digestive system, which is incredibly efficient at removing them.

Part of the way this works is that the fiber in the food we eat stimulates peristaltic action in the intestines, which moves everything through the intestines and colon, and out of the body. However, when we eat a diet deficient in fiber, peristaltic action is weak, and wastes can take a long time to get out.

By the way, do you know which three food groups central to the standard American diet have virtually no fiber? You guessed it: meat, dairy, and eggs.

ELECTROMAGNETIC ENERGY

In virtually every culture in the world there is a phrase that translates roughly as "You are what you eat." This kind of universal consistency might make us pause and consider the truth of this saying. We have already mentioned how the enzymes, pH, oxygen, water, and fiber in what we eat make us what we are.

Another major factor that contributes to our makeup is what is known as electromagnetic energy. We are electromagnetic creatures — there is actually an electromagnetic charge to our bodies. In fact, there is a kind of photography, called Kirlian photography, that can capture an image of electromagnetic charges. So if you take a Kirlian picture of my hand, you will see a sort of rainbow effect around it. Take a picture of an apple, and you will see a rainbow effect around the apple. Now bake that apple at 200°F for twenty minutes and take another Kirlian photograph. Where there was once an expansive rainbow field, there will now be only a slight emanation from the apple. Its electromagnetic energy has been largely destroyed.

Which brings us back to "You are what you eat." If you eat food that is vibrant, alive, and full of energy, how do you think you will feel? Conversely, if you eat food that is cooked to death and devoid of living energy, how do you think you will feel? With every bite, it's your choice.

PREVENTING AND HEALING DIABETES WITH A RAW-FOOD DIET

RABBI GABRIEL COUSENS, MD, MD(H), Diplomat of the American Board of Holistic Medicine, and Director of the Tree of Life Rejuvenation Center

The pandemic of type 2 diabetes today stems from a complex imbalance in the body's metabolism of carbohydrate, protein, and fat. It results in a significantly accelerated aging process and a degeneration that may take between ten and nineteen years off one's life span. It kills one person every ten seconds. Although many people have a genetic susceptibility to type 2 diabetes, the true causes (which activate the genetic potential physiology of the disease) lie in the diet and lifestyle choices people make. That is, genetics loads the gun, but poor diet and lifestyle choices pull the trigger. In Ayurveda, we refer to unhealthy diet and lifestyle choices as "crimes against wisdom."

The good news is that type 2 diabetes is a curable disease, a fact that is common knowledge in the live-food community. The current belief systems taught in medical school and to the general public claim that type 1 and type 2 diabetes are irreversible and are an accelerated march toward death. And they are — if one stays with mainstream dietary and medical approaches. From my thirty-five years of research and clinical experience on the subject — which are summarized in my book *There Is a Cure for Diabetes* and dramatized in the movie *Simply Raw: Reversing Diabetes in 30 Days*, which was filmed at the Tree of Life Rejuvenation Center in Patagonia, Arizona — a clear and successful approach has emerged that we now offer in our Reversing Diabetes Naturally 21-Day Program. In this program, we have found that 30 percent of the classically diagnosed type 1 diabetics and 45 percent of the type 2 diabetics stop taking all their medications, including insulin, and reach a consistent healthy fasting blood sugar of less than 100. Also, their LDLs, inflammatory cytokines, and hypertension usually return to normal levels. There is usually a fifteen- to twenty-pound weight loss, with the record being forty-four pounds in the twenty-one days. These seemingly miraculous results have become rather commonplace.

The key factor in this natural reversal is that the participants follow a 100 percent live-food, plant-based, organic, high-mineral, high-enzyme, well-hydrated, low–glycemic index, low–insulin index, individualized diet in which they eat modestly. Until their values have stabilized and remained in a healthy range for three months, we do not even allow participants to eat fruits, grains, or beans. After the three months are completed, low-glycemic fruits and a small amount (20 percent of total caloric intake) of cooked foods may be added. We also like people to do moderate exercise, yoga asana, and meditation.

By eating a raw-food diet, diabetics can rapidly transform the misery of a diabetic physiology into the joy of a healthy physiology. The recipes in this book give a wonderful feeling of what this healing diet looks like. If even 2 percent of pre-diabetics and diabetics in the United States followed this approach, it would result in the healing of approximately 1.6 million people. The time has come for us to love ourselves enough to take action to heal ourselves. This book gives us the skills to do so.

Cooking denatures our foods, severely diminishing the protein, vitamins, and minerals available to our bodies. Most people today eat foods that have been treated with chemicals, pesticides, herbicides, fungicides, hormones, and preservatives and that have been irradiated, broiled, baked, fried, freeze-dried, stored on a shelf for a few years, or popped into a microwave. And they eat them expecting to be healthy. Wake up and smell the wheatgrass!

The health crisis we are experiencing today in the United States and other countries is largely a result of our food choices. As animals, we are part of nature. Eating highly processed, denatured, adulterated, and unnatural foods is going to have health repercussions. The good news is that when we give our bodies the living foods they were meant to have, they operate in optimal health.

Allow me to reiterate that at the center of a well-balanced raw vegan diet are green leafy vegetables and other chlorophyll-rich foods such as seaweed. These foods have an unsurpassed ability to deliver oxygen and alkalize the body due to their high mineral contents, and they are optimal for building an internal environment where fungi, mold, and parasites are hard-pressed to survive.

IMPORTANT NOTE: It is essential for vegans to supplement their diets with vitamin B_{12}. While B_{12} does exist in plant foods, there is no definitive research showing that the human body is able to absorb plant-based B_{12}, whereas animal sources of B_{12} are assimilable by the body. For this reason, all vegans should regularly supplement their diets with B_{12}. This is especially important for nursing vegan mothers because B_{12} is vital for proper development of a child's nervous system. Damages from B_{12} deficiencies are irreversible, so don't wait.

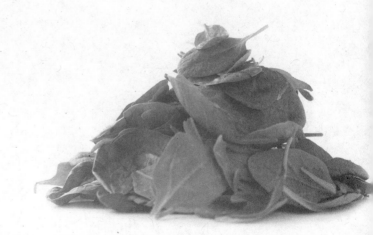

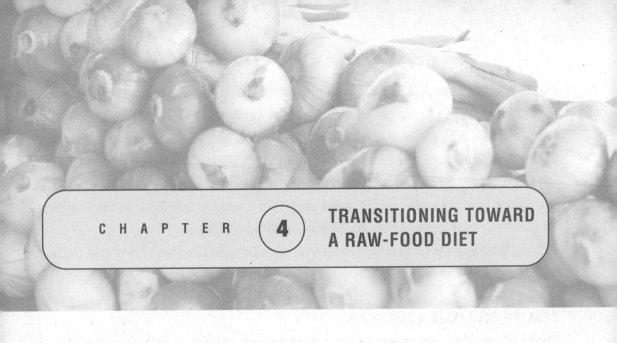

CHAPTER **4** TRANSITIONING TOWARD A RAW-FOOD DIET

I know there are a lot of readers who in a perfect world would be doing an hour of yoga every morning, meditating during lunch break, thinking only pure and grateful thoughts throughout the day, and eating a 100 percent raw, vegan, organic diet at all three meals. There is a tendency to want to make a resolution to "do it all" at once. And that might work for about .001 percent of you, but for the rest of us, it's more about incremental change.

What works best for most people is a steady, gradual, and gentle movement toward a healthier, happier you. Setting unreasonably ambitious goals is only setting yourself up for disappointment and disempowerment.

In diplomacy, steps toward resolution are referred to as "confidence-building measures." Since we'd all like to have more peace, it might be a good idea to think of our own progress this way: small, achievable steps that are doable and help create a momentum in the right direction.

So, how about ten minutes of yoga and stretching every morning? What about a fifteen-minute walk before you start your workday? Perhaps five minutes of meditation before you turn in at night (tuning in before you turn in).

Or how about one totally healthful meal each day? Or maybe set a goal of eating raw only five or six days a week, so you don't have to face the prospect of life without that Grand Slam breakfast! Start with something achievable. Breakfast, for example, is so doable. Wait till you get to the breakfast section — we have lots of delicious, easy-to-make recipes for you, including smoothies, oatmeal, and granola. Plus, you can make a smoothie any time you get hungry!

Once breakfast is conquered, adding in a salad for lunch is a breeze. You can even learn how to bump up that salad until it's a delicious and filling nutritional powerhouse — check out chapter 10, Making a Salad a Meal.

And then you are on to soups, desserts, dips, breads, crackers, and more. So have fun, and enjoy your food!

DEALING WITH FOOD ADDICTIONS

Those of us who have grown up on a contemporary Western diet have food addictions galore. I know I do. Fortunately, my three-year-old daughter does not. She has never eaten foods like refined flours and sugars, highly processed foods, meats, or dairy, all of which create negative addictions. We are helping our daughter create a very healthy and positive relationship with food.

But most of us were brought up with a less-than-optimal diet and a relationship to foods that includes an emotional attachment to eating them. We often have deep-seated and mostly unconscious feelings of giving ourselves a treat when we choose to eat many foods that we now know are far from optimal.

We can help the next generation by giving them a healthier start. But for the vast majority of us, we must begin by recognizing that we ourselves are food addicts — and not getting down on ourselves because of it! It simply is what it is, and now it is up to us to decide what to do about it.

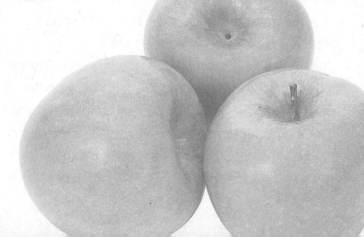

Many people who learn about the incredible benefits of raw and living foods try to use willpower to overcome their food addictions. While this will work for a while, usually willpower alone doesn't work in the long run. Instead, it's best to take the opportunity to become aware of our beliefs and attitudes about food, educate ourselves, and be loving and gentle with ourselves as we evolve toward a healthier relationship with food.

I will give you an example. There have been times I have really felt like having a piece of traditional baked pizza. This is not terribly surprising considering the fact that I grew up in an Italian American family, that my dad makes an incredible pizza, and that he also taught me how to make one at a young age. Consequently I have had an emotional attachment to pizza. So how do I handle the hankering?

When I first feel the desire for a slice, I usually think back to when I was giving up smoking many years ago. The trick was not to ask myself "Do I want to smoke a cigarette?" but to ask "Do I want to live life as a smoker?" A single cigarette is not going to significantly harm me. However, living life as a smoker would seriously compromise my health, as well as having many other negative effects on my life. And life as a smoker always begins with the next cigarette.

So, with food addictions I try to do the same thing, changing "Do I want to eat a piece of pizza?" to "Do I want to live life as a pizza eater?" While asking the second question, I envision a very round version of me eating pizza (as I mentioned, my last name, Rotondi, means "the round ones" in Italian). I really don't want to be round. I like being slim, light, and energized. So this thought often helps me get past the pizza hankering.

However, sometimes the hankering comes back — again and again. What to do? Use willpower to suppress my desire for pizza? If a desire for a specific food comes up repeatedly, I will go out and eat a small portion of that food. However, I will do it consciously. I will tune in to how my body feels before I eat the pizza and then focus on how the pizza smells, looks, and tastes. I will also be conscious of how I feel five minutes after I eat it, and thirty minutes, and an hour later. Usually what happens is that the first bite is okay but mildly unsatisfying. The second bite is really not a treat at all, and I realize that what I am eating tastes a bit like cardboard (keep in mind that when you eat a raw-food diet for any length of time, your taste buds change and cooked foods don't taste the same anymore). Then after five minutes I feel a heaviness in my stomach. After half an hour, I feel lethargic and already wish I hadn't eaten the pizza.

The point is that if we try to suppress all our cravings, in the end we get wound so tight that the spring may break and we might run out and eat three large pepperoni pizzas with extra cheese! It's better to get out of judgment mode and work on evolving our relationship with food. The more we exercise our body consciousness and really listen to our bodies, the more we will replace old food habits, thought patterns, and addictions.

By the way, if you have any other addictions in your life, moving to a raw-food diet can often help in kicking them as well. Once we can control the food we put in our mouths, everything else becomes easier.

DETOXING AND FASTING

In my experience, periodic detoxing and fasting can be a highly beneficial practice that leads to enhanced energy, minimized or eradicated disease, and a higher quality of life. I am not going to offer any set program for detoxing — that would require a whole book, because no one program works for everyone. But I do want to say that eating a raw-food diet is in itself a cleansing and healing process. So if you don't normally eat a high percentage of raw foods, doing so is like a form of fasting and will result in the aforementioned benefits.

If you do eat mostly raw, your body is already cleansing. You can expedite and deepen this process with periodic juice fasting. Green-juice fasting in particular is one of the best ways I know to detox and cleanse the body while still ensuring that you are getting the full gamut of necessary nutrients. (By the way, green juices also contain lots of minerals that help eliminate toxins released during a fast.) In fact, juicing can increase the amount of nutrition your body is able to absorb from food. Normally your digestive system has to pull nutrients out of the fiber in food as it passes through your intestines. Because juicing removes the fiber from foods, your body is able to get a much higher percentage of nutrients from the same food with less effort.

There are many detox programs now commercially available. Some of them are great. Many, however, take an aggressive approach, which causes your body to rid itself of toxins very quickly. While this might sound good, the results can be very uncomfortable and sometimes dangerous. The question is, What's the rush? I have often seen people get excited about cleaning out their bodies after having gone through long periods on a less-than-optimal diet. They get through their cleanse with great doses of willpower, then come off the detox too fast and start eating the same less-than-optimal diet as before — or even overindulge because of a built-up desire for "forbidden foods."

Again, rather than dramatic shifts in direction, I suggest incremental changes in your diet that you can maintain and even improve over time. This translates into gradually eating an increasingly raw diet.

To me, a cleanse or fast is time we take out of our lives to refocus our consciousness through contemplation, stillness, and loving ourselves. I think a gentle and loving fast is far better for most people in most situations than an aggressive and dramatic one. While an aggressive fast might appeal more to our desire to "do it all," one of the underlying benefits of fasting is to let go of some of the "doing" and allow ourselves to just be.

By the way, if you are just getting started with raw foods, juice fasting is an excellent way to clear the way and prepare your body for a new, healthier chapter.

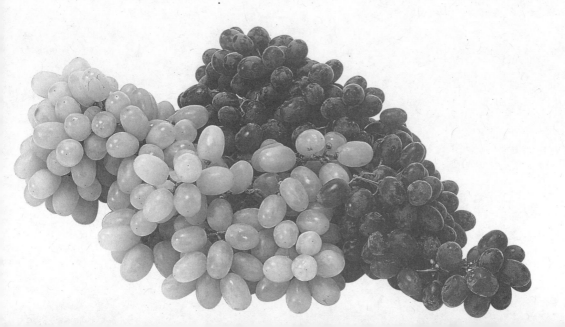

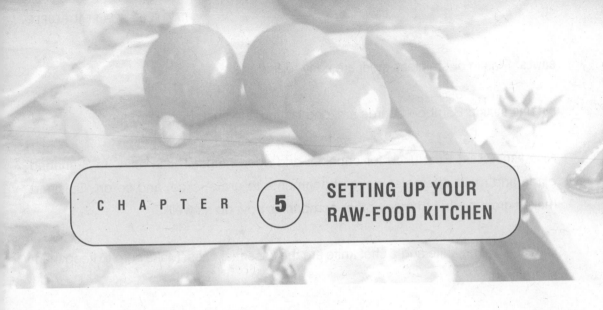

If you have a knife and a cutting board, you are ready to start. Well, you don't really need a cutting board. And even a sharp stick will get you started.

The point is, don't think you can't do this because you don't have the cash to invest or enough space for the equipment. Raw-food cuisine is based primarily on chopping up vegetables and fruits and sprouting grains, seeds, and nuts and dehydrating them. This cuisine was practiced for millions of years by our far less technologically endowed forebears. Now we have blenders, juicers, and food processors to save time.

But start with what you've got. Here is some information about some of the equipment, utensils, and gadgets that are helpful in setting up a raw-food kitchen. Many of these items are available at www.leaforganics.com.

BASIC EQUIPMENT

BLENDER: Best used for sauces, dressings, and creams. A high-speed blender with a manual speed control is best. I use mostly Vitamix blenders, but there are others, such as Blendtec, that are great as well. And keep in mind that any blender will be good to start with, even if it isn't high powered or fancy. I used my grandmother's old punch-button-speed-control blender for a long while. And you are virtually guaranteed to find a used blender or food processor at any garage sale. I used to buy them for a couple of bucks apiece and give them to friends.

BOWLS: Plastic or stainless steel are easy to find.

CUTTING BOARD: Bamboo boards are long lasting and sustainably produced.

FOOD PROCESSOR: Best used for chunkier and drier things. These have an S-shaped blade and most often also have attachments to grate, slice, and so on. Cuisinart makes great ones, but many other companies now do as well.

KNIVES: A paring knife and a chef knife are the essential ones. Make sure to keep them sharpened.

STRAINER: A double-screen strainer is best and longest lasting.

GOOD TO HAVE
  Dehydrator
  Juicer
  Salad spinner
  Spiral slicer (a machine that cuts vegetables and fruits into very thin, ribbonlike
      slices; Saldacco is one good brand)

STOCKING YOUR PANTRY
You don't need to have a ton of food on hand, but stock enough for day-to-day snacking, and remember that the more you have on hand, the more room you'll have for creativity.

Also remember that the first law of raw-food preparation is

Don't wait until you are hungry to make your food!

Here are some commonly used ingredients in raw-food cuisine to keep in your kitchen. Don't worry if you don't have all of them. You can always add ingredients one recipe at a time.

HERBS AND SPICES: **FRESH:** It's almost always best to use fresh! I love cilantro, dill, parsley, basil, oregano, and thyme.
DRIED: Some of my favorites are cayenne pepper, cinnamon, cumin, curry powder, and nutmeg.

LEGUMES: Chickpeas, lentils, and mung beans, all great sources of protein.

NUTS: My faves are almonds, Brazil nuts, hazelnuts, pine nuts, and walnuts — all great for snacking or for use in recipes. And some nut butter is always good to have on hand — anything tastes good with nut butter on it!

OILS: Coconut, olive, and sesame seed oil (make sure all are cold pressed and organic).

PRODUCE: **FLAVORING STAPLES:** Garlic, ginger, and onions. (I use lots of these!)
FRUITS: Apples, blueberries, durians, goji berries, lemons, mangoes, oranges, papayas, pineapples, strawberries, tomatoes, etc.
GREENS: There are so many to choose from — keep trying new ones. My favorites are arugula, collard greens, dandelions, kale, mesclun greens, and spinach.
SPROUTS: Alfalfa, broccoli, onion, sunflower, etc.
VEGGIES: Avocados, bell peppers, broccoli, cabbage, carrots, cauliflower, celery, cucumber, etc.

SEA VEGGIES: Dulse (my favorite), Irish moss (great for making desserts thicken), kelp, nori sheets (great for roll ups), and wakame.

SEEDS: Flax, pumpkin, sesame, and sunflower; also, raw tahini (if it doesn't say raw, it probably isn't).

BE PREPARED

Here are some ideas for things to have ready and available, plus some general tips about preparing meals.

- Keep a bag of peeled ripe bananas in the freezer. This way you can always make a smoothie!

- Keep a huge salad in the fridge at all times. Fill it with such goodies as assorted greens, root vegetables such as carrots and beets, and fresh herbs. This allows you to grab a quick salad anytime or fill a wrap quickly.

- Make enough of your favorite salad dressing to last all week.

- Mix up a big batch of your favorite dip, such as hummus (page 100) or Cashew Kreme Cheeze (page 93), to which you can add different flavors to vary the taste throughout the week.

- Always keep some sprouts ready in your refrigerator. Sprouted sunflower seeds are especially easy to prepare and versatile, and they are a great addition to any salad.

- Keep some soaked nuts in the fridge — great for a sweet, crunchy snack, on salads, or for whipping up some nut milk. Soaked nuts will last 3 to 4 days in the fridge. Be sure to rinse them once a day to maintain freshness. Be alert for any signs of mold growing on them — this often shows up as little white spots.

HELPFUL HINTS FOR PREPARING RAW FOODS

If you are a competent cooked-food chef, you already have many of the basic skills necessary to be a raw-food chef. However, I will go over some important raw-food preparation techniques here.

Using Knives

Good knife skills are a great asset to have for raw-food preparation. I will teach you a couple of techniques here; be sure to practice them slowly and with great care.

The first law of using a knife is never to cut toward yourself or any part of your body. Never! Always cut away from yourself. That way, if you slip or lose control of the knife, you are still safe.

The second law of using knives is to keep your knives sharp. It seems slightly counterintuitive, but a dull knife is a dangerous knife because you have to use more force than you would have to employ with a sharp knife, and slip-ups are more likely to happen.

Also, while they are not essential, I like to use ceramic knives. They are incredibly sharp, and they don't leave any metal particles on the food, which can cause the food to spoil more quickly.

SLICING AND CHOPPING: I have seen people use all kinds of funny techniques for slicing. The one I learned in Paris as a teenager has worked well for me over the years. I suggest you start with something easy like a celery stalk.

Hold a knife in one hand and the celery stalk on a cutting board with your other hand, with your thumb on one side and your pinky, ring finger, and middle finger on the other. This gives you a stable platform. Next, bend your index finger back and point the tip down the stalk. The first knuckle of your index finger will be extended slightly, giving you a surface to rest your knife blade against. Slice downward. Then slide your index finger back slightly and slice again. You will be able to control the thickness of the slices by how far you bring back your index finger. You will occasionally move the whole "platform" of the three fingers and thumb backward as well. Start this very slowly.

Many people think of chopping as an up-and-down motion. But my favorite chopping technique actually involves rolling the knife back and forth. Many chef knives have rounded blades to make this easier.

Start by holding a knife in your preferred hand with just the tip touching the board. Then bring the knife handle downward, causing the blade to roll down the board from its tip to its heel. Then raise the knife handle back to your starting position, rolling the blade back up along the board. This technique is much easier to control than a straight up-and-down motion, as the knife is always in contact with the board.

DICING: There is a trick for dicing quickly and efficiently. I learned this in Paris as a way to dice onions quickly to avoid eye irritation. Though we're using an onion as an example, the same approach works for most round fruits or vegetables you want to dice, such as tomatoes, oranges, jicama, and so on.

First, cut off the ends of the onion and peel off the outer skin. Then make two to four vertical slices in the onion (from top to bottom), cutting almost all the way down to the bottom, but not quite (if it's not cut all the way through, the onion doesn't fall into pieces). Turn the onion 90 degrees and repeat. Now you have an onion with a grid of slices in it but that's still in one piece. Roll the onion onto its side so the cuts are from right to left (or left to right). Hold the onion as for slicing above, and starting with the cut side, slice downward, working your way into the onion and toward the uncut end of it. The result is diced onions. The final piece of onion that was not sliced at first can then be cut and diced separately in a jiffy.

Cutting Corn

It's amazing how delicious corn is uncooked, straight off the cob! If you want to remove the kernels from an ear of corn, first husk the corn. Then, with one hand holding your knife and the other holding the corn vertically with the bottom end against a cutting board or the bottom of a large bowl, slice downward along the length of the ear. Try to get as many of the kernels as possible without cutting into the inedible cob. Because you need a strong purchase on the corn with your free hand, you will probably be able to slice off only about two-thirds of the kernels in one direction. Then, turn the ear upside down and slice off the last third.

Opening Coconuts

I was first shown how to open a coconut by a little ten-year-old boy on a tiny island off the coast of Tanzania. When you crack open a coconut, the pristine white meat and clear water present themselves. When you do this in a hot, dry place such as Tanzania, the world seems magical indeed.

I recommend that you use young green coconuts in these recipes. In supermarkets, you sometimes come across hard, brown, bark-like coconuts. These are more mature coconuts best for their thick and very flavorful meat, which is great for grating. The young green coconuts are usually husked before they're shipped to supermarkets, so they look white instead of green.

There are a variety of techniques for opening coconuts. I will teach you my favorite because it is also the safest and most elegant. It leaves a perfect round hole on the top of the coconut, and this hole makes it easy to spoon out the meat once you have removed the water.

Hold the coconut on its side with your left hand (reverse for lefties, please). Using a sharp chef's knife or butcher's cleaver in your right hand, slice the husk off the top of the coconut. Do this by putting the weight of your right shoulder over the coconut and pushing down on the knife. Keep on turning the coconut with your left hand and then slicing down with the knife until the pointy top of the coconut has been shaved down to the shell. Then stand the coconut up with the shaved end on top and grasp its side with your left hand, keeping your fingers well out of the way. (No fingers near the top!) With the knife in your right hand, slice down into the outside of the shaved top of the coconut, piercing it. Then just crack the top of the coconut open by using the knife as a lever. The first time you try this it can be a bit intimidating, but it will soon be as easy as opening a bottle.

Either drink the coconut water immediately or pour it into a glass or bowl. To remove the coconut meat, insert the handle of a spoon between the coconut shell and the meat and run it around the rim, separating the meat from the shell. Keep on working your way around, deeper and deeper, until you have the whole chunk of coconut meat separated in one piece. Alternatively, using a chef's knife or a butcher's cleaver, you can chop the coconut in half and then just use a spoon to carefully scoop out the meat in pieces as large as possible.

Preparing Lemons

The best way to peel a lemon or other citrus fruit is to first slice away the ends so it is more stable for cutting. Then, cut away the peel, leaving as much of the white pith as possible. (The pith contains bioflavonoids, which are great for your health, and it also helps make sauces lighter and fluffier.) A quick way to juice a lemon is to cut it in half, then cup one half in one hand with the cut side out, insert a fork into it, and squeeze the lemon while turning the fork and lemon in opposite directions. To eliminate seeds, simply squeeze into a sieve over a bowl (or just juice the lemon into a bowl and remove the seeds with a fork).

Whenever making any kind of sauce or dip in a blender using lemons, limes, or oranges, always put them in before the other ingredients, at the bottom of the blender. The citrus will be the first to get processed and will create the juices that help move the rest of the ingredients around and get well blended.

One discovers innumerable little techniques and methodologies when making raw foods. In the following chapters I will share the ones I have learned as I teach you how to make specific recipes.

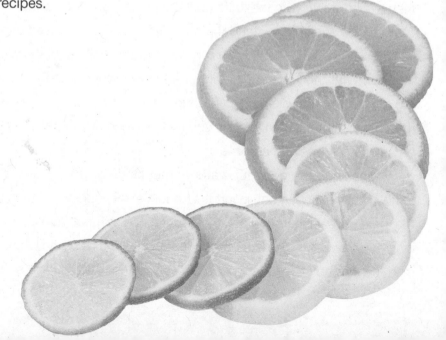

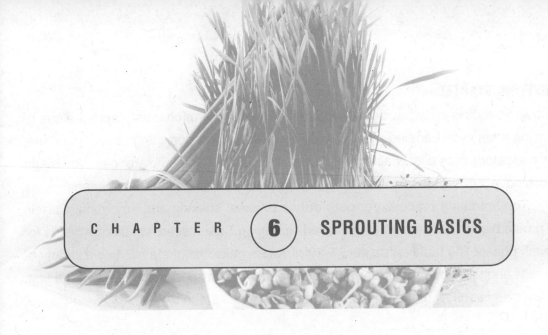

CHAPTER 6   SPROUTING BASICS

Sprouts are nature's little nutritional powerhouses. Here's why: Every seed is endowed with a large reserve of energy and nutrients to fuel its growth until it can derive enough energy from its external environment. Once the seed has germinated, enzymes in the seed trigger the conversion of the stored nutrients from a dormant to an active and bioavailable state, making the nutrients available for the seed's growth. So the seed becomes a sprout, and eventually the sprout becomes a plant, once it has used up all the initial stored energy of the seed and is able to draw energy from its environment. By eating sprouts, humans are able to access this energy and nutrition for themselves. These concentrated sources of living energy are delicious and easy to digest, and many varieties are high in protein. For much more on the health benefits of eating sprouts, check out *The Sprouter's Handbook* by Edward Cairney.

There are lots of different kinds of special sprouting equipment out there, some of which can be really useful. But the truth is that most sprouting can be done very simply without any special equipment. For many sprouts, a jar, a bucket, or even a bowl will work. Some smaller seeds, such as alfalfa, clover, or onion, can also be sprouted in a bag; hemp bags are often used for this purpose.

GETTING STARTED

Buying seeds is easy nowadays, and they're extremely affordable. There are lots of online stores you can find by simply doing a search for "sprouting seeds." Our site, www.leaforganics.com, has some excellent seeds at competitive prices. You might also have a co-op or specialty store in your area that carries sprouting seeds.

The sprouting process consists of two phases: soaking and sprouting. Certain sprouts benefit from a third stage called "greening." Each seed has unique needs for each phase. The table on pages 57–59 provides guidelines for sprouting a variety of seeds and tells you specifically what is needed for each seed in each phase. But first, here's an overview of the phases.

SOAKING: During this first phase, the seeds are immersed in water and simply soak. This washes off the enzymatic growth inhibitor that coats many seeds and nuts. The reason they have this inhibitor is to ensure that if the seed or nut falls to the ground into a single drop of water, it won't immediately start to sprout and then die for lack of moisture. The growth inhibitor needs to be completely dissolved to signal the seed that it is safe and moist enough to germinate. And that is what this first phase is all about — germinating the seed, grain, or nut.

For this phase, you simply place the seeds, grains, or nuts in a jar, bucket, or other receptacle and immerse them in water over a length of time. Covering the receptacle with a screen, towel, or cheesecloth will ensure that no dust or bugs can get in, while still allowing air to pass through.

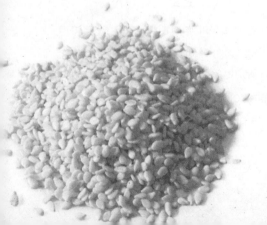

As you can see from the "Quantity" and "Yield" columns of the sprouting chart, there is often a big difference between the quantity of seeds you start with and the amount of sprouts you end up with. For instance, chickpeas grow from 1 cup to 3 cups during the process. For this reason, when you are preparing to soak your seeds, be sure to choose a receptacle that is big enough to accommodate the amount of sprouts indicated in the yield column; you want to give your seeds space to grow without overflowing the receptacle. While the seeds are soaking, store the receptacle at room temperature and out of direct sunlight. If it gets too hot, mold can grow, and if it's too cold, the sprouting process will take longer.

The time period for soaking depends on the seed. The third column of the chart gives you a range of time for this soaking phase. As a rule of thumb, if the seed has an extended soaking phase (more than twelve hours), the water should be changed and the seeds rinsed at least once every twelve hours. Some seeds, such as buckwheat, have special rinsing needs during the soaking phase; these are explained in the "Rinsing Guidelines and Additional Comments" column.

SPROUTING: Once the seed has germinated in the soaking period, you pour the water out, rinse the seeds, and repeat until the water pouring out is clear and clean. After the final rinse, return the seeds to their receptacle. At this point, you do *not* immerse the seeds in water. The time period for each seed's sprouting period is given in the "Sprouting Time" column of the chart. During this period, the seeds are growing and need to be rinsed periodically to keep them clean, fresh, and sweet. As with the soaking phase, the rule of thumb is to rinse them at least every twelve hours while they're sprouting. Specific rinsing requirements during the sprouting stage are given in the "Rinsing Guidelines and Additional Comments" column.

Another rule of thumb is that when the "tail" of the sprout is as long as the seed, it has optimally sprouted. Follow the timing instructions in the chart, but you will often have to use your own judgment because different seeds will sprout differently depending on environmental variables such as humidity and temperature. You can taste and chew the sprouts to try to determine if they are fully sprouted. Generally, optimally sprouted seeds are soft and a little sweet. If they sprout for too long, they become stringy and hard.

GREENING: Some seeds have a third and final stage known as "greening." Greening means taking the fully grown sprout and placing it in sunlight for an hour or so. This allows the sprouts to use photosynthesis to produce chlorophyll in their leaves, creating beautiful and nutritious green leaves. Usually, indirect light is best for this phase. Be careful not to "cook" the sprouts with too much direct light or heat. The chart indicates which sprouts you'll want to green.

Once the sprouts have reached their optimal length, put them in the refrigerator. This restricts or ends the sprouting process. Nevertheless, the finished sprouts should still be rinsed one or two times a day while stored in the fridge. Try to use them as soon as possible after they reach optimal sprouting. Most sprouts will last at least two or three days in the fridge. Some, such as lentils, can last even longer, but my advice is to sprout them for when you need them. They are always best when they are most fresh!

A WORD ABOUT NUTS

Unlike seeds and grains, nuts are usually soaked but not sprouted. With nuts, the important thing is that the enzymatic coating gets washed off and the nutrients become more bioavailable, and soaking takes care of that. Also, nuts are already soft enough to eat without being sprouted, as opposed to most seeds and grains, which are still pretty hard after the initial soak.

However, if you soak nuts, you end up with moist, soft nuts, which are not always what we want for recipes or just for snacking. A common practice is to soak nuts and then to drain and dehydrate them. This process delivers nuts in their optimal nutritional state but with a nice, dry, crunchy consistency and more flavor. It is not essential to soak and then dehydrate nuts, but if you are looking for peak nutrition, this is the way to do it. Throughout this book, I have specified when nuts should be soaked before being used in a recipe. If I haven't indicated that they be soaked, then you can use either unsoaked nuts or nuts that have been soaked and then dehydrated.

SEED, GRAIN, OR NUT	QUANTITY	SOAKING TIME	SPROUTING TIME	RINSING GUIDELINES AND ADDITIONAL COMMENTS	YIELD
ADZUKI BEAN	1 cup	12–14 hours	3–5 days	Rinse 2 or 3 times daily.	8 cups
ALFALFA	3 tablespoons	5 hours	4–6 days	Rinse every 12 hours. "Green" by putting in indirect sunlight for about one hour when fully sprouted.	4 cups
ALMOND	6 cups	8–10 hours	2 days	Usually used soaked only; if you do sprout them, rinse every 12 hours. Both can be stored in the fridge for 4–6 days if you change the water daily.	8 cups
AMARANTH	2 cups	3–5 hours	2–3 days	Rinse at least 3 times daily.	6 cups
BARLEY (HULLED)	2 cups	6 hours	24 hours	Rinse 2 times while sprouting.	5 cups
BROCCOLI	3 tablespoons	8 hours	3–4 days	Rinse 2 or 3 times daily. "Green" by putting in indirect sunlight for about one hour after fully sprouted.	3 cups
BUCKWHEAT (HULLED)	2 cups	6 hours or longer	1–2 days	Rinse every 4 to 8 hours during both soaking and sprouting phases.	4 cups
CHICKPEA (GARBANZO BEAN)	1 cup	18–24 hours	2–3 days	Rinse 2 or 3 times daily.	3 cups
CLOVER	6 tablespoons	5 hours	4–6 days	Rinse every 12 hours. "Green" by putting in indirect sunlight for about one hour after fully sprouted.	6–8 cups

SEED, GRAIN, OR NUT	QUANTITY	SOAKING TIME	SPROUTING TIME	RINSING GUIDELINES AND ADDITIONAL COMMENTS	YIELD
FLAX	1 cup	1 hour	n/a	Generally used soaked only. Will soak up a large amount of water during the soaking phase, so be sure to add enough.	2 cups
LENTIL	1 cup	8 hours	2–3 days	Rinse 2 times daily. Keeps well in fridge once sprouted.	4 cups
MILLET	1 cup	6–10 hours	12–24 hours	Sprouts quickly. Rinse and drain every 8–12 hours.	3 cups
OAT GROAT (HULLED)	1 cup	8–10 hours	1–2 days	Rinse 3 times daily.	1 cup
ONION	1 tablespoon	4–6 hours	4 days	Rinse 3 times daily.	2 cups
PEA	1 cup	8–12 hours	2–3 days	Rinse every 12 hours. Keeps well in fridge once sprouted.	2½ cups
PINTO BEAN	1 cup	12 hours	3–4 days	Rinse 4 times daily.	3–4 cups
QUINOA	1 cup	3–4 hours	2–3 days	Rinse well before soaking. Rinse every 12 hours while sprouting.	3 cups
RADISH	3 tablespoons	6–12 hours	3–5 days	Rinse every 8–12 hours. "Green" by putting in indirect sunlight for about one hour after fully sprouted.	3–4 cups
RYE	1 cup	6–8 hours	2–3 days	Rinse 2 times daily.	3 cups
SESAME (HULLED)	1 cup	8 hours	n/a	Used soaked only. Can be used for tahini.	1½ cups
SESAME (UNHULLED)	1 cup	4–6 hours	1–2 days	Rinse 4 times daily.	1½ cups

SEED, GRAIN, OR NUT	QUANTITY	SOAKING TIME	SPROUTING TIME	RINSING GUIDELINES AND ADDITIONAL COMMENTS	YIELD
SPELT	1 cup	6 hours	1–2 days	Rinse every 12 hours.	1½ cups
SUNFLOWER (HULLED)	1 cup	6–8 hours	1 day	Remove skins from top of water when soaking.	2 cups
TEFF	1 cup	3–4 hours	1–2 days	Rinse every 12 hours. Smallest grain and highest in protein.	2½–3 cups
WHEAT	1 cup	8–12 hours	2–3 days	Rinse every 8–12 hours.	2–3 cups
WILD RICE	1 cup	3 days	n/a	Most wild rices don't actually sprout but split open. There is some controversy whether wild rice is truly raw.	3 cups

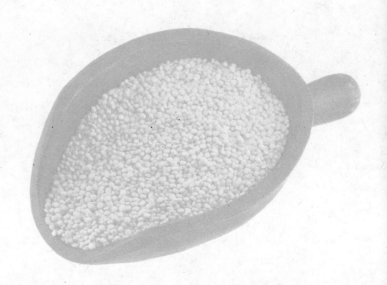

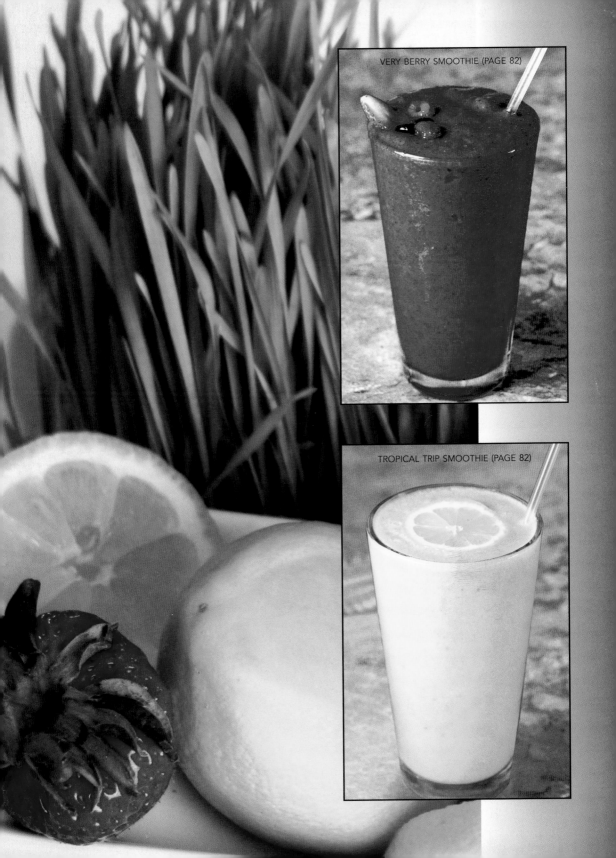

VERY BERRY SMOOTHIE (PAGE 82)

TROPICAL TRIP SMOOTHIE (PAGE 82)

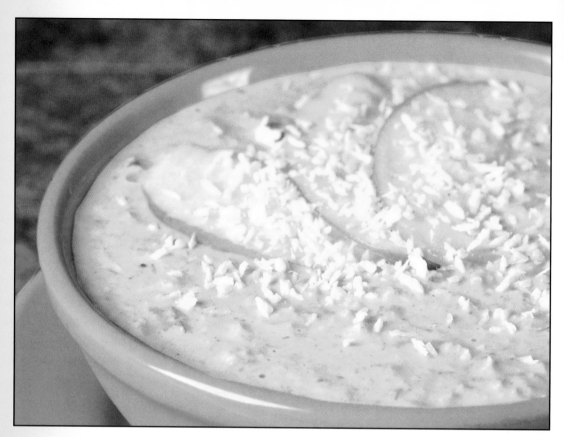

REAL DEAL OATMEAL (PAGES 83–84)

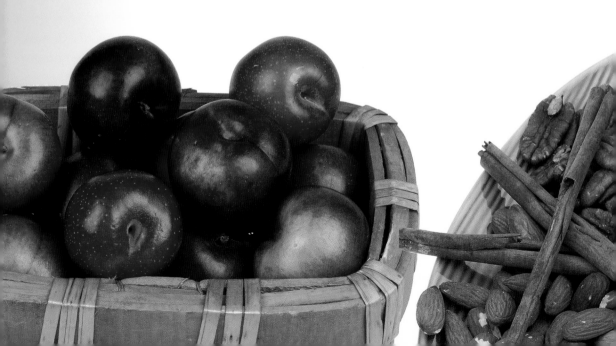

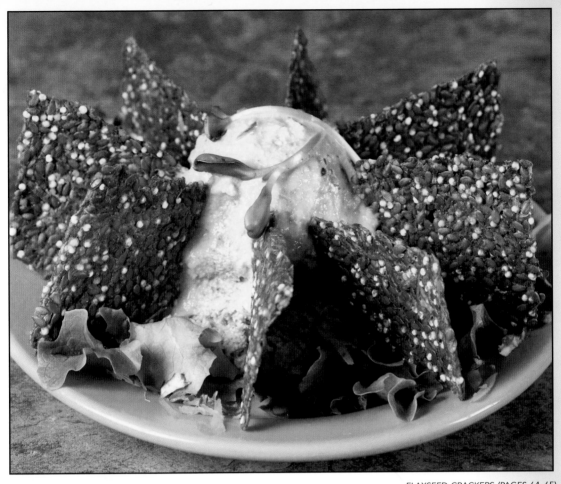

FLAXSEED CRACKERS (PAGES 64–65)
WITH SPROUTED CHICKPEA HUMMUS (PAGES 100–101)

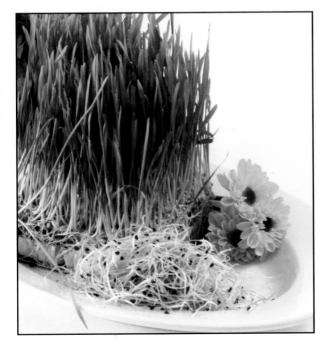

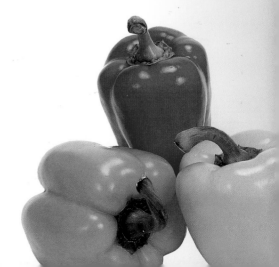

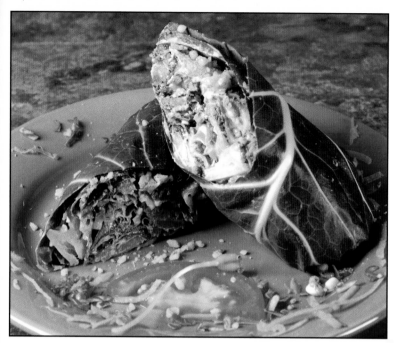

CAESAR IN THE RAW WRAP (PAGE 108)
NORI ROLLS WITH ATLANTIS PÂTÉ (PAGES 89–90)

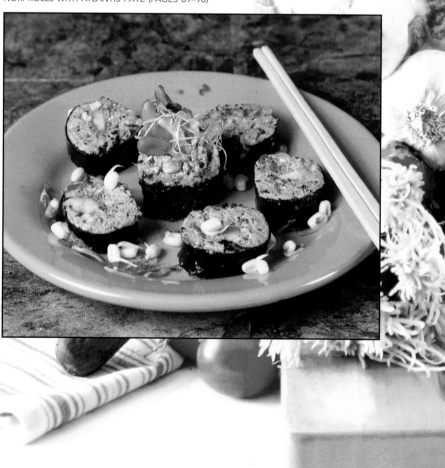

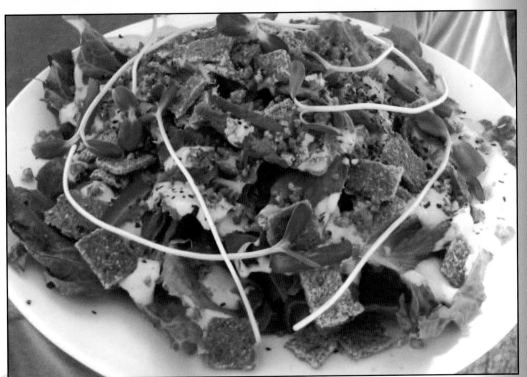

CAESAR IN THE RAW SALAD (PAGES 107–8)

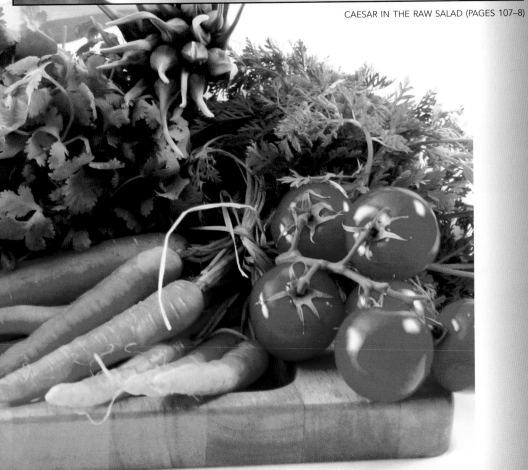

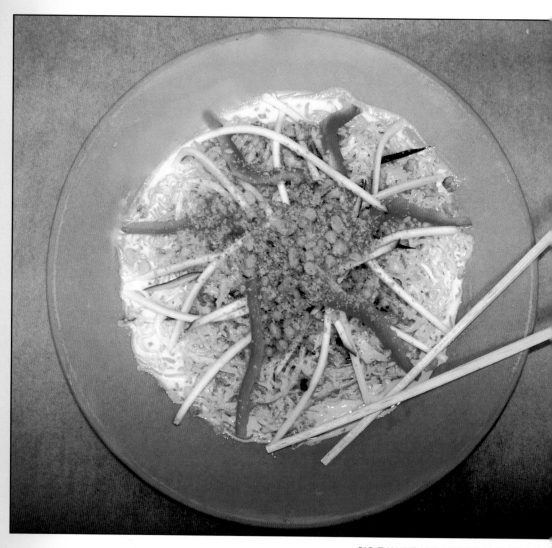

PAD THAI WITH KELP NOODLES (PAGES 132–3

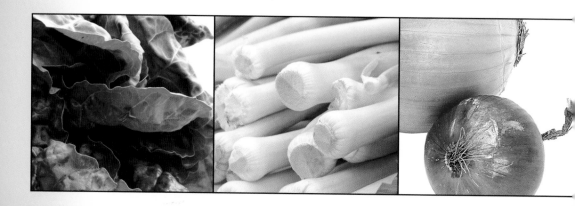

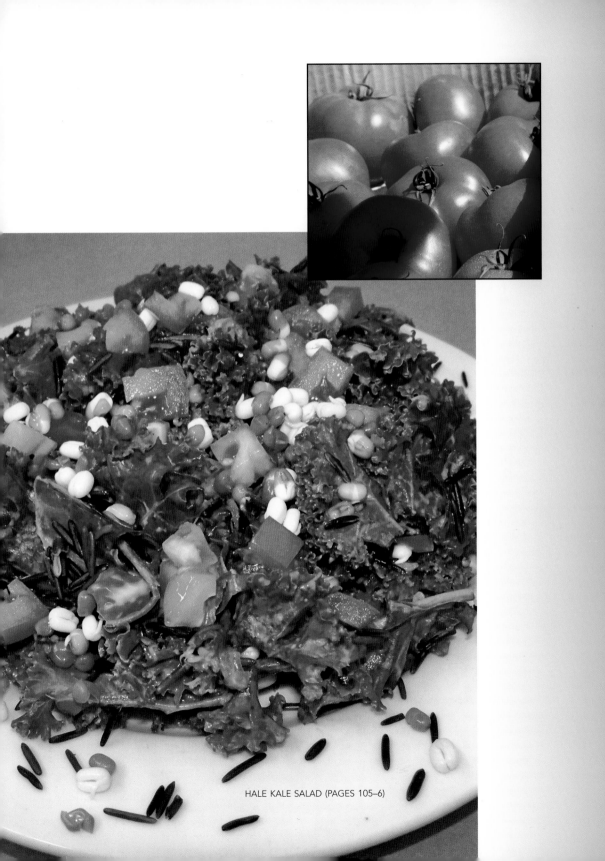

HALE KALE SALAD (PAGES 105–6)

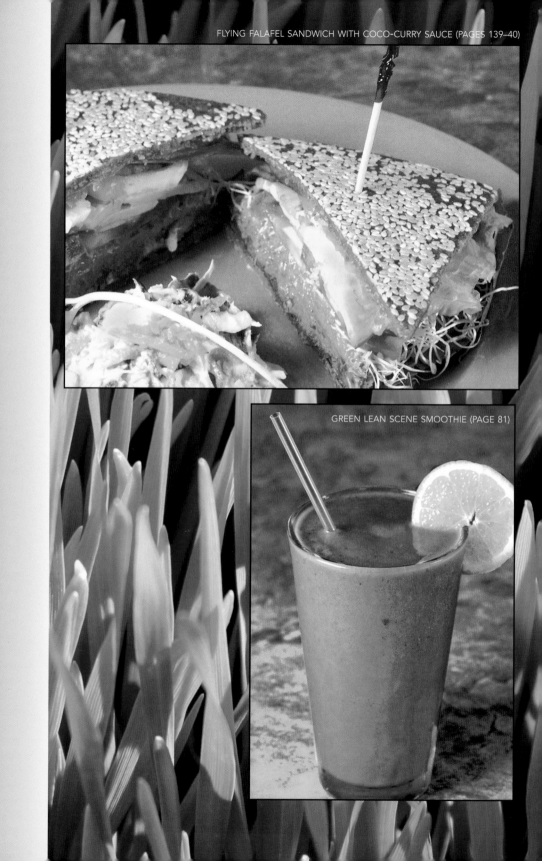

FLYING FALAFEL SANDWICH WITH COCO-CURRY SAUCE (PAGES 139–40)

GREEN LEAN SCENE SMOOTHIE (PAGE 81)

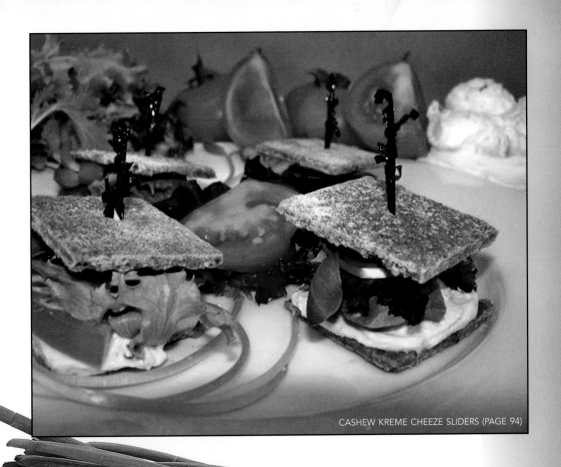

CASHEW KREME CHEEZE SLIDERS (PAGE 94)

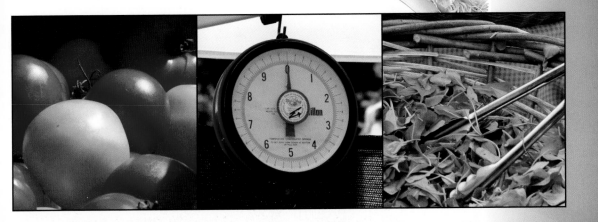

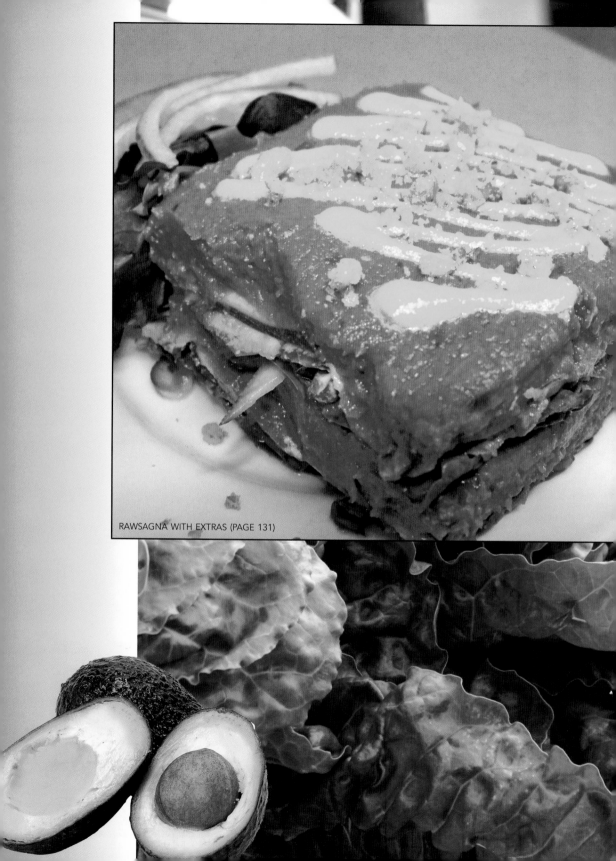

RAWSAGNA WITH EXTRAS (PAGE 131)

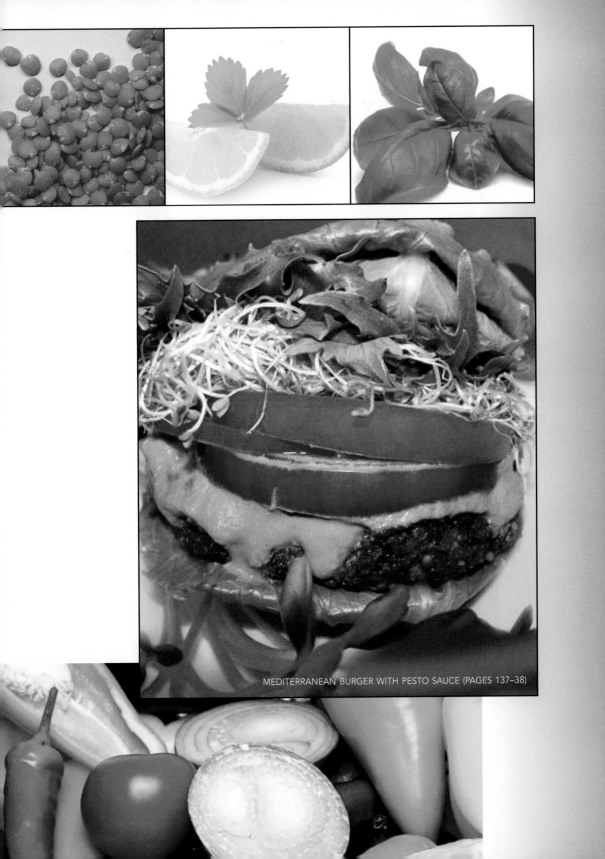

MEDITERRANEAN BURGER WITH PESTO SAUCE (PAGES 137–38)

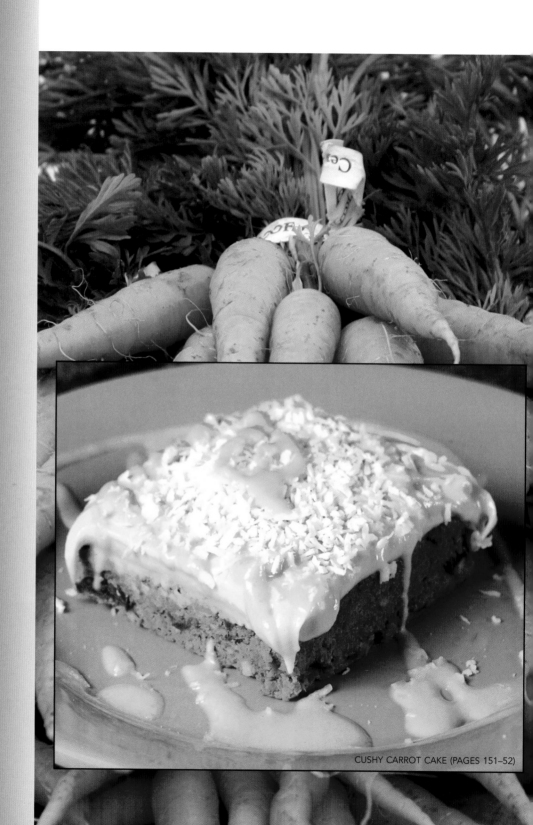

CUSHY CARROT CAKE (PAGES 151–52)

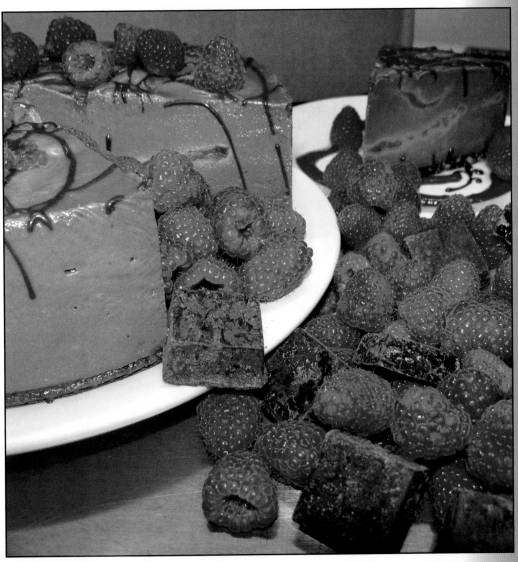

RASPBERRY CACAO CHEEZECAKE (PAGE 150)

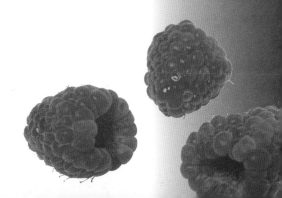

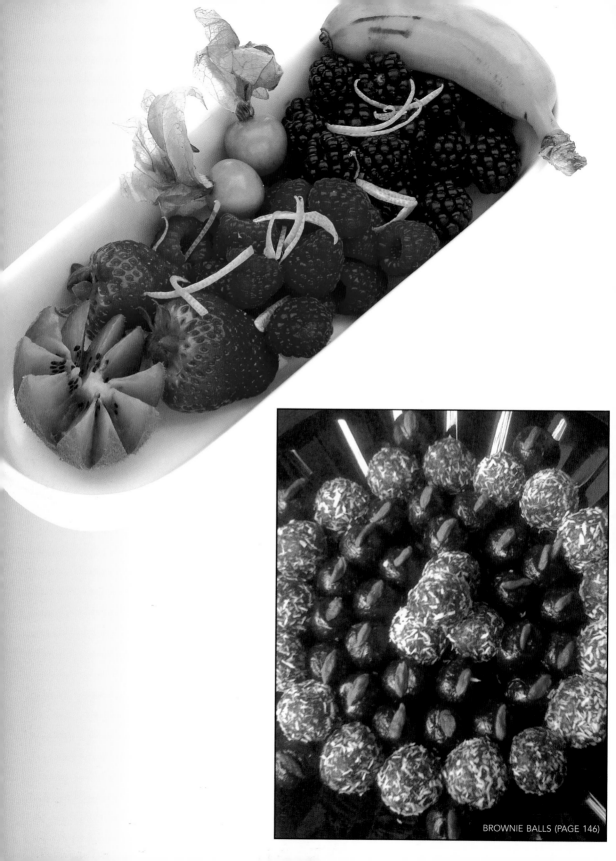

BROWNIE BALLS (PAGE 146)

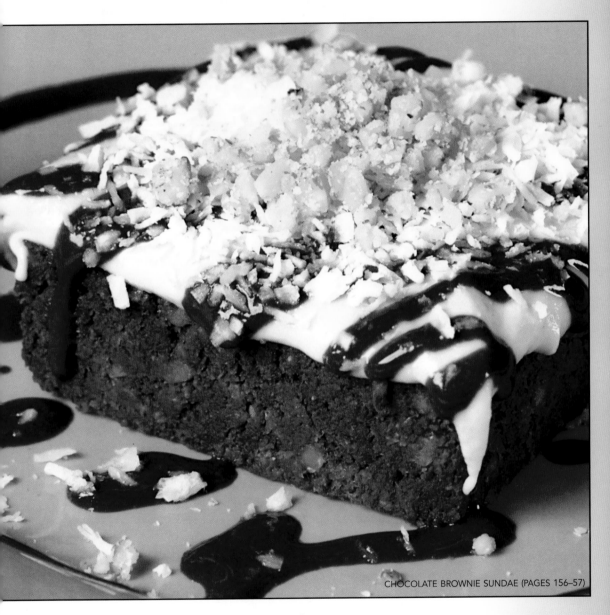

CHOCOLATE BROWNIE SUNDAE (PAGES 156–57)

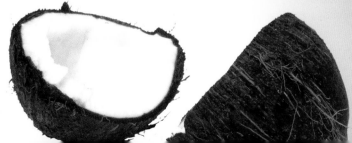

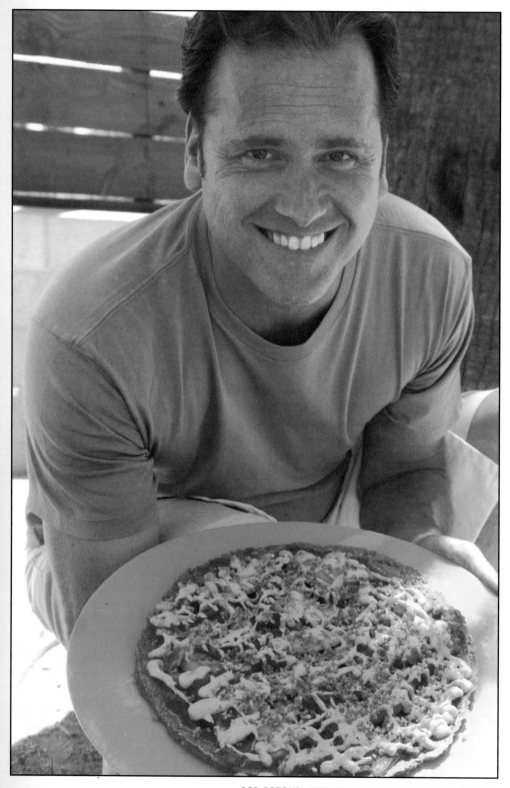

ROD ROTONDI WITH PIZZA PIZZAZZ ABBONDANZA (PAGE 72)

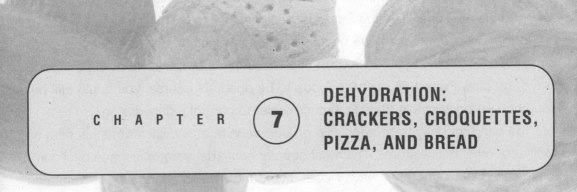

CHAPTER (7) DEHYDRATION: CRACKERS, CROQUETTES, PIZZA, AND BREAD

I lived for nearly seven years in a Bedouin village in the Sinai Desert. When I first arrived, there were no phones, paved roads, or electricity lines. I learned from the Bedouin people a lot about living simply. I also learned about their food. One of the most interesting things I learned was the age-old tradition of dehydrating food.

Because of their nomadic lifestyle, the Bedouin needed food that would travel. So they would form hummus into little patties and put the patties out on a rock in the sun. By the end of the day, the hummus had dehydrated and was golden brown and crispy on the outside and warm and yummy on the inside. And they could take this food with them as they traveled.

This very same process has been used by people around the world to preserve foods. This process also has the benefit of maintaining food's key digestive enzymes and is a cornerstone of raw-food preparation. While it is possible to prepare raw foods without dehydration, the process results in crispier textures and denser foods that pack in nutrition. Dehydration is especially useful for preserving foods and for transitioning to a raw-food diet.

Each of the following chapters addresses a different area of raw-food preparation. Since almost all of them include recipes that call for dehydration, we are going to start with this chapter. However, if you don't have a dehydrator yet or you find dehydration too complex or time-consuming at this point, please just skip this chapter for now and go on to the next one, "Getting Started: Breakfast."

In the raw-food kitchen, we use a very simple machine called a dehydrator to simulate the effects of sun and warm air. It is simply a box that holds slide-in food trays and blows warm air over the foods to be dried. Of course, you could still put food outside on a rock in the sun, but it's easier to control a dehydrator!

You can find dehydrators for sale on our website at www.leaforganics.com as well as at other online stores. The most popular home dehydrator is made by a company called Excalibur. They have three-, five-, and nine-tray models. I recommend the nine-tray model because it has the same footprint as the five-tray but is more versatile. Because dehydration creates a longer shelf life for food, you usually will want to make larger batches, so having a larger dehydrator is convenient.

Choose a dehydrator with both a temperature control and a timer — a temperature control is essential, and having a timer makes it more convenient. Most dehydration for raw foods is done at around 110°F. Since food enzymes die at 118°F, 110°F is a safe temperature to dehydrate at. In some cases, when there is a significant mass of food being dehydrated and it is quite moist (such as with croquettes or burgers), the temperature can be raised for the first 30 to 60 minutes to up to 120°F or even 130°F. This is because lots of evaporation actually cools the food. Once the moisture level (and thus the rate of evaporation) drops, you should bring the temperature down to 110°F or less.

The dehydrator tray is made up of two essential pieces and an optional third piece. First is the basic frame of the tray. Often these are plastic, but in some cases they are stainless steel mesh. Next is the plastic grid, which sits on top of the tray frame. The plastic mesh has small holes for air to pass through. When the food you're dehydrating is relatively dry (nuts, for example), you place it right on the plastic grid.

On the other hand, when the food you're dehydrating is wet, if you were to put it directly on the plastic grid, it would sink into the grid, drip down, or congeal and stick to the grid, and you would have to break it apart to remove it. To avoid this problem, you place a ParraFlex sheet (the optional part of the dehydrator tray) on top of the plastic mesh and set the food on the ParraFlex sheet. ParraFlex is a reusable, lightweight, flexible, nonstick material that works perfectly as the dehydration surface for wet or sticky foods (such as most bread and cracker doughs, as well as some fruits).

Once the wet food you have placed on the ParraFlex sheet has dried out some, it can be flipped onto a tray without a ParraFlex sheet. The original tray can then be removed and the ParraFlex sheet peeled off the food, so that the food can then dehydrate from both sides; this technique is explained in detail in the Flaxseed Crackers recipe (pages 64–65). ParraFlex sheets are usually sold separately, so you'll need to order them with your dehydrator.

By the way, conventional ovens don't normally make good dehydrators. First of all, most ovens won't hold a temperature as low as 110°F, and second, some airflow is needed to remove the moisture from the air. Some convection ovens might work in that regard, but again, it's hard to hold a temperature low enough, so a dehydrator is called for.

CRACKERS

One of the beauties of dehydration is that it allows us to create food with solid and crispy textures. Crackers are great because they last a long time without refrigeration and can be used as a base for dips. You'll see that the quantity of crackers from each recipe varies, depending how thinly or thickly you spread the dough. If you spread the dough thickly, you'll get fewer crackers.

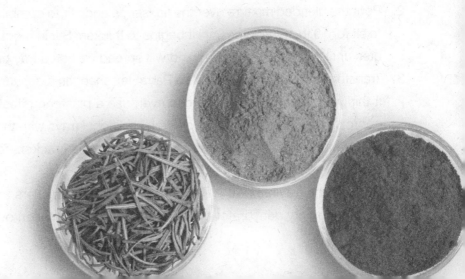

FLAXSEED CRACKERS

This is one of the most popular types of raw crackers. Flaxseeds have a property that makes them ideal for making crackers. When soaked in water, they become viscous, and then when they're dried, they become crispy.

Makes 60 to 80 crackers

1¾ cups flaxseeds (brown, golden, or mixed)
1 medium carrot, chopped (about ½ cup)
4 one-inch pieces fresh ginger, peeled and minced (about ¼ cup)
3 medium cloves fresh garlic, minced
½ teaspoon cayenne pepper
½ cup nama shoyu (substitute tamari or ⅓ cup miso paste to make gluten free)
Dash of curry powder
Dash of ground cumin
3 tablespoons cold-pressed olive oil
1 bunch fresh cilantro leaves, chopped (about 1 cup)
4 cups water, plus additional (up to 1 cup) as needed

1. Put the flaxseeds in a large bowl. Combine all the other ingredients with the 4 cups water in a blender and blend well.
2. Pour the blended mixture over the flaxseeds and stir to combine. Allow the mixture to sit for 10 to 15 minutes until it begins to thicken. Stir in more water every 15 minutes until the mixture is goopy and will spread well on a tray but is not too runny.
3. Transfer 2 cups of the mixture to a ParraFlex sheet on a dehydrator tray and spread it thinly with a spatula (or you can even use a plastering float or trowel) until it is approximately ¼ inch thick. Repeat on additional trays with the remaining mixture.
4. Put the trays in the dehydrator and dehydrate the crackers for 3 to 4 hours, until the tops are dried.
5. Remove the trays from the dehydrator. To flip the crackers to dry the other side, place an empty dehydrator tray (without a ParraFlex sheet) over the top of one of

the cracker trays, hold them both together, and flip them. Then remove the top dehydrator tray and peel the ParraFlex sheet off the crackers. Repeat with the other trays. Put the crackers back into the dehydrator and dry until crispy, 6 to 8 hours.

SICILIAN SAVORY SNAPS

This is one of the best dipping crackers ever. It's got a nice oniony, Italian herb flavor with a mellow background created by the sunflower seeds.

Makes 100 to 120 crackers

1 cup ground flaxseeds
3 cups ground sesame seeds
1¾ cups ground sunflower seeds
3 cups sprouted oat groats (see chart, page 58), ground
2 medium carrots, roughly chopped (about 1 cup)
3 medium onions, roughly chopped (about 3 cups)
1 teaspoon ground cinnamon
½ tsp ground nutmeg
1 tablespoon fresh oregano
1 teaspoon sea salt
3 cups water
3 tablespoons agave nectar

1. In a large bowl, combine the ground flaxseeds, sesame seeds, and sunflower seeds with the oat groats.
2. Put the remaining ingredients in a food processor and process well.
3. Add the mixture from the food processor to the dry ingredients and blend well.
4. Spread on sheets and dehydrate as with the Flaxseed Crackers (previous recipe).

CROQUETTES

Croquettes are veggie patties made with fresh veggies, fresh herbs and spices, and sprouted seeds, grains, and nuts, which are then formed into little balls and dehydrated at low temperature. I got the idea from falafels and then started experimenting, using different bases besides sprouted chickpeas. Stored in an airtight container in the fridge, they'll last ten days to two weeks, but as with all foods, they're best eaten fresh.

FLYING FALAFEL CROQUETTES

This is the raw and original falafel. No frying — that is, no carcinogens — needed! This is basically the same recipe as the one for hummus; the only difference is that we add ground seeds to the base. This adds dryness, nutrition, and heft to the falafel.

Makes 30 to 40 croquettes

5 cups sprouted chickpeas (see chart, page 57)
3 cups hulled sunflower seeds
2 medium lemons, peeled and quartered
½ cup tahini
6 medium cloves garlic
1½ bunches fresh parsley leaves (about 1½ cups)
3 tablespoons cold-pressed olive oil
1 tablespoon sea salt
2½ teaspoons ground cumin
1 cup coarsely chopped yellow onion

1. Put the sprouted chickpeas and sunflower seeds in a food processor and grind them well. Remove to a large bowl.
2. Put the lemons first, then all the other ingredients, in a blender and blend well.
3. Pour the blended mixture into the bowl with the chickpeas and mix well. Taste and adjust the seasonings.

4. Using an ice cream scoop or a spoon, scoop balls of the mixture onto a ParraFlex sheet on a dehydrator tray. You can make the balls anywhere from 1 to 2 inches in diameter. The larger they are, the longer they will take to dehydrate. Also, they can be in the form of patties instead of balls. Dehydrate at 125°F for the first hour. Then lower the dehydrator temperature to 110°F and dehydrate for another 9 to 13 hours, until they are golden brown and slightly crispy on the outside.

VEGGIE SUN BURGER CROQUETTES

Make a big batch of these, and you'll be able to plop them in a wrap, top off a salad, or just enjoy them as is for the next week. To create new recipes, simply change the sprouted seeds, veggies, and spices as you choose!

Makes 24 croquettes

½ cup hulled sunflower seeds
1½ cups flaxseeds
1 bunch fresh parsley leaves (about 1 cup)
3 small yellow onions, chopped (about 1½ cups)
3 medium cloves garlic
1 two-inch piece fresh ginger, peeled
6 to 8 ribs celery, chopped (about 3½ cups)
6 to 7 carrots, chopped (about 3 cups)
½ small head red cabbage, chopped (about 1½ cups)
2½ teaspoons sea salt
½ cup cold-pressed olive oil

1. Put the sunflower seeds in a blender and grind until powdery. Remove to a medium bowl.
2. Put the flaxseeds in a blender and grind until powdery. Remove to the bowl containing the sunflower seeds, and stir together.

3. Combine the rest of the ingredients in a food processor and process until well blended. Transfer to a large bowl, add the ground seeds, and mix well.

4. Using an ice cream scoop or a spoon, scoop balls of the mixture onto a dehydrator tray. Pierce each ball from the top with your finger, creating a hole in the middle but not all the way through, to accelerate dehydration. Dehydrate at 125°F for the first hour. Then lower the dehydrator temperature to 110°F and dehydrate for another 9 to 13 hours, until the croquettes are golden brown and slightly crispy on the outside. Store in the refrigerator.

Note: If the mixture ends up a bit wet so that it would seep into the spaces in the plastic grid of the dehydrator sheet, you will have to scoop the croquettes onto a ParraFlex sheet and then flip them after several hours, as with the Flaxseed Crackers (see recipes pages 64–65). However, I find I can often put these directly onto the plastic mesh on dehydrator trays.

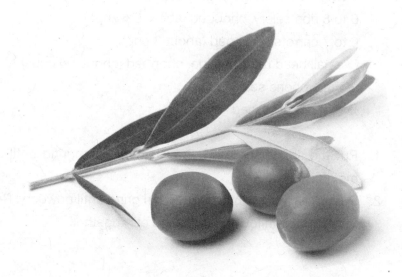

PIZZA

Some of my earliest memories are of my dad making food in the kitchen. He started teaching me to make pizza when I was only a few years old. He is a master with dough, and he taught me how to make it — even how to throw it up in the air on the back of my knuckles. (A nice trick, but a rolling pin ain't bad either.)

When I decided to make a raw pizza, I was determined to apply my dad's lessons and come up with a perfect pizza. I am really happy with the result and I hope you will be too.

The crust is critical. I have tasted raw pizzas out there that use lots of nuts in the crust. I think there is an overreliance on nuts in many raw-food recipes. Sure, nuts taste great, but that's largely because they are high in fat. They are great in the proper proportions, but don't overdo it.

Call me crazy, but I think that sprouted grains ought to be the base of a pizza crust. Nuts should be used sparingly (except perhaps in desserts, which is where we indulge a bit). So here is my recipe for a delicious and crispy pizza.

PIZZA PIZZAZZ

My dad explained that a truly great pizza always has three levels. First, the bottom of the crust should be crispy, so the first experience of biting into a slice should be the crispiness. The second level is a slight chewiness where the crispy crust blends with the topping to create a chewy middle ground. Finally, a warm and moist top finishes off the perfect pizza bite. All right, so let's start with the crust.

Makes 1 large pizza

For the Crust
1 small yellow summer squash, diced (about ½ cup)
4 to 5 medium carrots, chopped (about 2½ cups)
1 cup sprouted buckwheat (see chart, page 57)
½ cup sprouted sunflower seeds (see chart, page 59)

¾ cup sprouted lentils (see chart, page 58)

Dash of sea salt

¼ cup golden flaxseeds, ground

¼ cup soaked almonds (soaked 8 to 10 hours, drained, and rinsed)

⅛ cup diced yellow onion

For the Cheeze Sauce

⅛ cup chopped yellow onion

1 medium clove garlic

⅛ cup soaked pine nuts or macadamia nuts (soaked about 1 hour, drained, and rinsed)

¼ cup nutritional yeast

¼ cup mild miso paste

1 cup water, plus additional (up to ½ cup) as needed

1½ teaspoons turmeric

½ cup sprouted sunflower seeds

For the Marinara Sauce

¼ cup chopped yellow onion

2 to 3 medium cloves garlic

1½ cups chopped fresh tomatoes

1½ teaspoons fresh oregano leaves

4 fresh basil leaves

½ teaspoon sea salt

1 tablespoon cold-pressed olive oil

¼ cup sun-dried tomatoes, soaked 1 hour if not already soft

For the Rawmesan Cheeze

1 cup walnuts

1 tablespoon sea salt

½ cup nutritional yeast

Chopped basil leaves for garnishing

1. To make the crust: Put the squash and carrots in a food processor and blend well. Slowly add the remaining crust ingredients and continue to blend until the mixture reaches a doughlike consistency. (You may add herbs such as rosemary, tarragon, or basil, or sun-dried tomatoes or olives, for variety.)

2. Remove the dough to a ParraFlex sheet on a dehydrator tray and spread it evenly to a thickness of about ¼ inch.

3. Dehydrate for 4 to 5 hours, then flip by placing another tray (without a ParraFlex sheet) on top and inverting the crust onto the new tray. Remove the ParraFlex sheet, return the crust to the dehydrator, and continue to dehydrate for another 4 hours.

4. To make the Cheeze Sauce: Put all the ingredients except the sunflower seeds in a blender and blend well. Add the sunflower seeds slowly while blending, adding more water as needed to achieve a melted-cheese consistency.

5. To make the Marinara Sauce: Put all the ingredients in a food processor and pulse until you have a nice chunky sauce. Remove half the sauce to a bowl. Blend the remaining sauce until it reaches a smooth consistency. Add the blended sauce to the chunky sauce and mix well. Your sauce should have a perfect texture — smooth but with real chunks.

6. To make the Rawmesan Cheeze: Finely chop the walnuts with a knife or process them in a food processor, and put them in a medium bowl. Add the sea salt and nutritional yeast, and mix well. That's all there is to it.

7. To assemble the pizza: Generously spread the Marinara Sauce evenly over the crust; the sauce layer should be about ¼ inch thick. Top with the Cheeze Sauce (using a squeeze bottle is easiest) and garnish with chopped basil and Rawmesan Cheeze.

8. Put the pizza back in the dehydrator for about 30 minutes to warm it up. The 30-minute warm-up also allows the top part of the crust to marinate in the Marinara Sauce, which softens it and makes it a little chewy. This way, we end up with a crisp bottom of the crust, the softer, chewy top part of the crust, and the warm, gooey, and yummy topping — perfetto! Remove from the dehydrator and serve. Buon appetito!

VARIATIONS

Pizza Pizzazz Abbondanza

Before adding the Cheeze Sauce, add any number of toppings you like, such as sliced avocados, soaked sun-dried tomatoes, or marinated onions.

Italian Croutons

Okay, this is a cheap trick, I admit it, but I am keeping it simple! Make a couple of flats of pizza crust and cut them into crouton-sized pieces before flipping. Finish dehydrating and voilà! — croutons. Or you can call them "little snacky things." Put them out in a bowl and watch them disappear.

Italian Herb Bread

This is possibly an even cheaper trick — but this pizza crust also makes wonderful bread slices. Follow the recipe for the crust, but add some chopped fresh oregano, basil, and thyme while processing the dough. After dehydrating, cut the crust into bread slice–sized pieces and make sandwiches, or spread with guacamole. Try using different combinations of sprouted grains, seeds, veggies, herbs, and spices to make different variations.

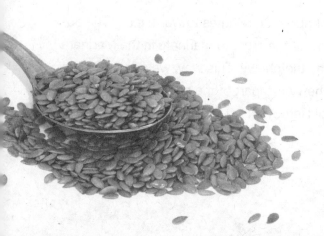

BREADS

As I mentioned earlier, the first breads were not baked. People sprouted the grains and then dehydrated the dough in the sun, creating delicious and incredibly nutritious bread. If you read J. R. R. Tolkien's Lord of the Rings books, you'll recall the magical bread created by the elves. It lasted incredibly long and was incredibly sustaining. Yep, elves are raw foodists.

MANGO BREAD

This is a nice chewy and slightly sweet bread, great to serve with so many things or on its own.

Makes about 24 pieces

2½ cups ground sesame seeds
1½ cups ground sunflower seeds
1 cup ground flaxseeds
1½ cups chopped fresh mango
1½ cups sprouted oat groats (see chart, page 58)
4 to 5 medium carrots, chopped (about 2½ cups)
½ teaspoon ground cinnamon
½ teaspoon ground nutmeg
1½ teaspoons sea salt
¼ cup agave nectar
1 cup water, plus additional (up to 1 cup) as needed

1. Put the ground sesame seeds, sunflower seeds, and flaxseeds in a large bowl.
2. Put the rest of the ingredients in a food processor and blend until smooth; add more water as needed to keep it all moving in the processor. If it stops blending, add a little more water, stir, and try again. Repeat until the mixture blends continuously.

3. Add the blended ingredients to the ground seeds and stir until evenly blended.

4. Remove the dough to a ParraFlex sheet on a dehydrator tray and spread evenly to a thickness of about ¼ inch.

5. Dehydrate for 3 to 5 hours, until the top of the dough is dry, then flip by placing another tray (without a ParraFlex sheet) on top and inverting the bread onto the new tray. Remove the ParraFlex sheet, return the bread to the dehydrator, and continue to dehydrate for another 10 to 12 hours, until dry but still flexible. Cut into 4-inch-square slices.

ARTISAN HERB BREAD

Sandwiches, anyone? This bread is especially good with any Mediterranean-inspired spread or sauce.

Makes about 20 pieces

¾ cup coarsely chopped yellow squash
1 medium carrot, shredded (about ½ cup)
1½ cups sprouted buckwheat
¾ cup sprouted sunflower seeds
¾ cup sprouted lentils
½ cup soaked almonds (soaked 8 to 10 hours, drained, and rinsed)
¼ cup coarsely chopped yellow onion
1½ teaspoons sea salt
1 cup water, plus additional (up to 1 cup) as needed
½ cup ground golden flaxseeds

1. Put the squash, carrot, buckwheat, sunflower seeds, lentils, almonds, onion, salt, and 1 cup water in a food processor and blend until smooth; add a little more water as needed to keep it all moving in the processor. If it stops blending, then add a bit more water, stir, and try again. Repeat until it blends continuously.

2. Put the ground flaxseeds in a large bowl. Add the blended ingredients to the ground seeds and stir until evenly blended.

3. Remove the dough to a ParraFlex sheet on a dehydrator tray and spread evenly to a thickness of about ¼ inch.

4. Dehydrate for 3 to 5 hours, until the top of the bread is dry, then flip by placing another tray (without a ParraFlex sheet) on top and inverting the bread onto the new tray. Remove the ParraFlex sheet, return the bread to the dehydrator, and continue to dehydrate for another 10 to 12 hours, until the bread is dry but still flexible. Cut into 4-inch-square slices.

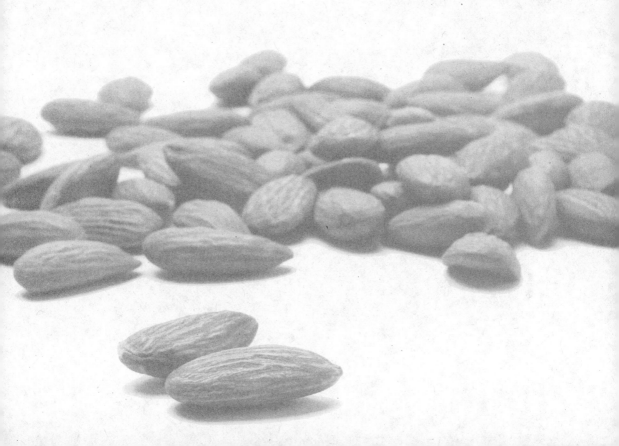

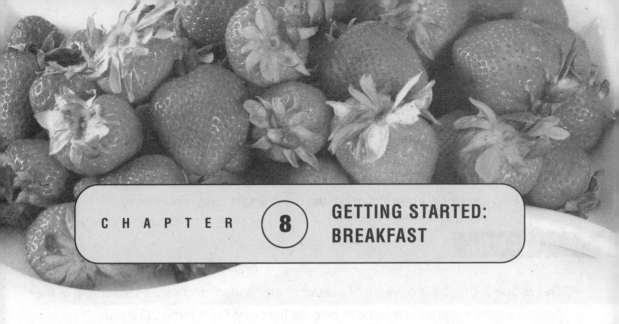

Good morning, Rawmerica! Ouch, that's bad. Talk about waking up on the wrong side of the bed. Let's try that again.

It's a beautiful day, and today we are going to add beautiful, delicious, all-natural, and fresh foods to our body temple. So let's start with breakfast!

In my experience, starting the day on the right note with a delicious, healthy, and nutritious breakfast sets me up for a great day, so our first objective is to do just that. I would like to add one more qualifier: it's got to be quick! Mornings are often the most rushed part of the day, so a healthy and quick breakfast is where we are heading.

Instead of focusing on what we might eliminate from our diet, let's focus on the positive: eating truly nutritious foods throughout the day.

SMOOTHIES

These days many places offer blended "nutrition drinks," but often they lack taste or actual nutrition. I want to teach you to make incredibly delicious, nutritious, and infinitely customizable smoothies that blow the fast-food options out of the water. The possibilities are endless in terms of both nutrition and taste. Also, keep in mind that kids love smoothies. My daughter is partial to the Virgin Piña Colada, although she just calls it a "white smoothie." She also likes "pink smoothies" (with strawberries) and "green smoothies" (with spirulina).

Smoothies start with a base liquid. Many on the market use highly processed mixes and have a years-long shelf life. These are less than optimally nutritious, and we can do better.

For starters we'll learn how to make simple nut mylk, which we can use to make many kinds of smoothies. These mylks, while nondairy, are creamy and delicious and full of living enzymes, essential minerals, healthy fats, and other nutrients.

NUT MYLK

This recipe is the result of years of research, meditation, and soul searching. It is the perfect base for smoothies but can also be the base for "kreme of" soups.

Makes 6 cups

1 cup nuts (your favorites)
6 cups water

1. Combine the nuts and water in a blender or food processor. Blend well.
2. Transfer to a pitcher and refrigerate. May be kept in the fridge for 2 to 3 days or until it separates or starts to smell funky.

Hope I didn't lose anyone with that one. Try it and you will be amazed at how such a simple recipe can make such a delicious drink! What you get is a frothy white milk with a nutty taste.

The higher the fat content of the nuts you use, the creamier your nut mylk will be. So macadamias or cashews will give you a creamier nut mylk than, say, almonds or hazelnuts. And the higher the ratio of nuts to liquid, the thicker the mylk will be. So the two factors affecting the richness and thickness of the mylk are the fat content of the nut and the ratio of water to nuts. Using fatty nuts and only a little water, you can actually make something as thick and delicious as frosting! Just add some dates or raisins for sweetness.

You can improve the nutritional content of the mylk as well as its taste by soaking the nuts for several hours before using them. Most nuts have enzyme inhibitors covering them that may be hard to digest. Simply soaking them for a few hours will remove this inhibitor and will make the nut easier to blend and digest. The easiest way to do this is, before you go to bed at night, to put a cup or two of nuts in a bowl of water and leave them on the counter overnight to soak. In the morning, pour off the water from the bowl. Depending on what kind of nut you are using, the water will probably be brownish tinged and bitter tasting. Rinse the nuts well until the water you pour off is clear and has no odor.

After you have blended the soaked nuts with water, you can put the nut mylk through a sieve or cheesecloth to remove any grit that remains. Personally, I often don't screen my mylks at home, but some people prefer a totally creamy texture. By the way, the nut grit that you remove can be used as a nice nutty filler to make cookies, breads, or a host of other treats.

You can also use coconut mylk instead of nut mylk to make smoothies. It's especially good as the base for tropical fruit smoothies. The recipe for coconut mylk is simple, as you'll see below.

COCONUT MYLK

Fresh young coconut meat makes a tastier mylk, but dried (at low temperature) works fine if you can't readily get fresh. Keep in mind that this recipe makes the simplest coconut mylk possible. You can add vanilla, agave nectar, spices, and other sweeteners to give the mylk more flavor. Coconut mylk is also good for making coconut curry sauces and coconut lassis.

Makes 6 cups

Meat of 1 small fresh young coconut (about 1 cup) or ¾ cup dried coconut flakes
6 cups water

1. Combine the coconut and water in a blender or food processor. Blend well.

To make smoothies, once you have your nut or coconut mylk, just add your favorite fruits. A number of smoothie recipes follow to get you started, but it really just comes down to adding whichever fruits you love — mangoes, bananas, blueberries, whatever! You can base your smoothie ingredients on what's available seasonally and locally.

So, with a few cups of nut or coconut mylk in the blender, add your fruit, and if you like your smoothies sweet, add some raisins, dates, agave nectar, yacon syrup, or some other healthy sweetener. Then blend — yummy!

It's a good idea to keep a bag of peeled ripe bananas and other fruits in your freezer. This gives you lots of flexibility with flavors, and adding a frozen banana makes smoothies nice and cold and thick.

You also can take your smoothie one step further and add in superfoods such as maca root powder (great for vitality and balancing hormones), spirulina powder (chock-full of chlorophyll and minerals), tocotrienol powder (high in vitamin E — great for hair and skin), raw cacao (high in antioxidants, and it gives you a boost!), hemp protein powder (high in protein, minerals, and good fats), and many more. Just blend these in with the rest of the ingredients. All these items should be available at your local health-food store, or you can order them online (try our website, www.leaforganics.com).

If you're in a hurry, you don't even need to make the nut or coconut mylk separately. You actually can just throw nuts, water, fruit, sweeteners, and superfoods together in the blender at the same time and blend. You also can use fresh-squeezed fruit juice instead of mylk, if you prefer.

So, there you have it — an infinitely customizable and nutritious breakfast in a snap. You can take it with you or sip it as you balance in tree pose or breathe slowly in deep meditation.

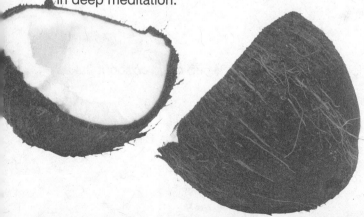

Here are a bunch of smoothie recipes we use at our restaurants. Try them, and then feel free to make up your own!

SMOOTHIE RECIPES

Each makes 1 sixteen-ounce smoothie

Berry Refreshing

⅓ cup blueberries

⅓ cup strawberries

⅓ cup raspberries

1 teaspoon agave nectar

1¼ cups Coconut Mylk

Blueberry Bonanza

1 medium banana

3 to 4 medium dates, pitted

¾ cup blueberries

1¼ cups Nut Mylk

Chocolate Milk

1 medium banana

3 to 4 medium dates, pitted

1 tablespoon cacao powder (or nibs)

1 tablespoon carob powder

1¼ cups Nut Mylk

Green Lean Scene

1 medium banana

¾ cup mango

3 to 4 whole kale leaves

½ teaspoon ground cinnamon

1¼ cups orange juice

Immuno Blastoff

1 medium banana

1 inch-and-a-half-long piece fresh
  ginger

½ medium lemon, peeled

½ medium apple, cored

3 to 4 medium dates, pitted

1¼ cups water

Mudslide Slim

1½ medium bananas

3 to 4 medium dates, pitted

1¼ cups Nut Mylk

Nutter Butter Naner Choco Coco

½ cup Brazil nuts

1 medium banana

1 tablespoon cacao powder

1 teaspoon carob powder

1 teaspoon maca powder

1 tablespoon agave nectar

2 to 3 medium dates, pitted

1 cup fresh coconut meat or ½ cup
  grated coconut

1¼ cups water

Protein Dream

1 medium banana

2 to 3 medium dates, pitted

3 tablespoons sprouted buckwheat

¾ cup strawberries

1¼ cups Nut Mylk

Raspberries and Kreme

1 medium banana

3 to 4 medium dates, pitted

¾ cup raspberries

1¼ cups Nut Mylk

Tropical Trip

1 medium banana

2 to 3 medium dates, pitted

¾ cup tropical fruit, such as mango,
    pineapple, or papaya

1¼ cups Coconut Mylk

Very Berry

1 medium banana

¼ cup raspberries

¼ cup strawberries

¼ cup blueberries

½ medium apple, cored

2 to 3 medium dates, pitted

1¼ cups water

Virgin Piña Colada

Water and meat of 1 young coconut

1 cup chopped pineapple

1 banana

Bee pollen, green powder, or protein
    powder (optional)

The Works

¼ cup strawberries

¼ cup blueberries

¼ cup raspberries

¼ cup tropical fruit, such as mango,
    pineapple, or papaya

3 medium dates, pitted

1 tablespoon hemp protein powder

1 tablespoon flaxseed oil

1 teaspoon cacao powder

1 teaspoon maca powder

1 teaspoon tocotrienol powder

¾ cups Nut Mylk

½ cup Coconut Mylk

PORRIDGES: OATMEAL AND BUCKWHEAT

If you're feeling like having a more solid breakfast to sustain you for a longer period of time, it's hard to beat a porridge. Oatmeal is incredibly delicious and filling — it's a real substantial meal. Many people eat oatmeal because of its reputation for being heart friendly and healthy in general. What people often don't realize is that the oatmeal most people eat is a grossly inferior version of what it can be. Most oatmeal is made from oats that have been steamed and pressed before they are cooked. Often they come in little paper sachets and last on a shelf for years, and you just add hot water and stir. I am going to teach you to make the real deal — oatmeal from sprouted oats — plus a couple of porridges with buckwheat, another healthy and satisfying breakfast grain.

REAL DEAL OATMEAL

You must use oat groats for this recipe. The flat little white oat wafers most people use to make oatmeal are not oat groats. Even steel-cut oats are not oat groats. Oat groats look like fat brown grains of rice. You can soak them overnight and make them in the morning, but it's best to give them another twelve to twenty-four hours to sprout and soften before you make oatmeal, unless you like it a bit chewy.

Serves 4 to 6

4 cups soaked and sprouted oat groats (see chart, page 58)
1½ tablespoons almond butter
1½ medium bananas
¾ cup raisins (soaked 1 hour and drained)
1 tablespoon ground cinnamon
1 tablespoon water
½ teaspoon nutmeg
¾ cup agave nectar
1 medium apple, cored and grated (about 1 cup)
Sliced apples and dried shredded coconut for garnishing (optional)

1. Put all the ingredients except the grated apple and garnishes in a food processor
    and blend well. It's always nice to have multiple textures and consistencies in
    your food, so one trick for achieving this is to process the mixture a little, then stop
    and remove half of it to a medium bowl. Then blend the rest well, and combine
    the two mixtures in the bowl. This creates a creamy base with a little chunkiness.
2. Stir the grated apples into the mixture, garnish with apples and coconut if you like,
    and you're ready to eat!

VARIATIONS

To take this up a notch, you can add all kinds of superfoods and other supplements to
your oatmeal to make it even more nutritious and delicious. Here is the recipe for one
of my favorite superfood-supplemented oatmeals, and another that not only is nutritious
and delicious but also helps wake you up. For those trying to avoid gluten (oat groats
do contain some), you can make a delicious sprouted buckwheat porridge instead.

Emerald City Oatmeal

Follow the directions for regular oatmeal, then stir in 1 teaspoon spirulina powder
and 1 tablespoon flaxseed oil.

Count Choco Maca Oatmeal

Follow the directions for regular oatmeal, then stir in 1 tablespoon cacao powder and
1 teaspoon maca powder.

Living Buckwheat Porridge

Follow the directions for regular oatmeal, but substitute 2 cups soaked and sprouted
buckwheat (see chart, page 57) for the oat groats. To give this a different great taste,
try substituting ½ cup yacon syrup for the agave nectar.

Fruity Oatmeal or Buckwheat Porridge

To make a fruity version of oatmeal or buckwheat porridge, slice up some fresh fruit
and add it over the top, or mix it in. Peaches, mangoes, blueberries, strawberries,
and many other fruits work very well.

BUCKWHEAT BREAKFAST FEAST

This is a wonderful, gluten-free breakfast treat that can be modified endlessly depending on seasonal availability of fruits and nuts. My three-year-old daughter, Lilli, loves it. We like to decorate it with the sliced fruit to make it more colorful and fun for her.

Serves 4

2 cups sprouted buckwheat (see chart, page 57)
1 avocado, peeled and pitted
Pinch of sea salt
1½ cups fresh fruit (your favorites, such as sliced peaches, mangoes, strawberries, or blueberries)
½ cup chopped walnuts or pecans for garnishing

1. Combine the buckwheat sprouts, avocado, and a pinch of salt in a food processor and process until it reaches an oatmeal-like consistency.
2. Remove to a serving dish and top with fresh fruit. Garnish with chopped walnuts or pecans and serve.

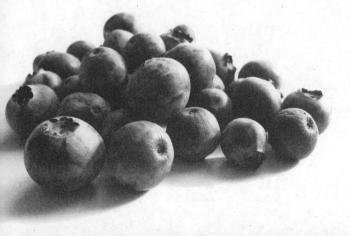

GRANOLA

Granola is another great breakfast item. You can eat it as is or top it with a nice nut mylk. It's also a great snack food to carry around and munch on when you are hungry.

GROOVY GRANOLA

Here is an easy-to-make recipe that is incredibly delicious. Serve it with Nut Mylk (see recipe, page 78), and you'll be in granola heaven!

Makes 5 cups

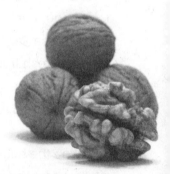

4 cups sprouted buckwheat (see chart, page 57)
½ cup walnuts (soaked 2 hours, drained, and rinsed)
½ cup raisins
½ cup agave nectar
4 teaspoons ground cinnamon

1. Put the sprouted buckwheat in a large bowl. Add the walnuts and raisins and mix well.
2. In a blender, mix together the agave nectar and cinnamon. Pour over the buck-wheat mixture and mix well.
3. Spread the mixture on dehydrator trays with ParraFlex sheets on top, and place in the dehydrator for 4 to 6 hours, or until crunchy. If it sticks together, break it up into granola-sized clumps.

VARIATIONS

Very Berry Granola

Follow the directions for regular granola. After the dehydration step, mix in ½ cup dried blueberries, ½ cup dried strawberries, and ½ cup dried raspberries.

Tropical Granola

Follow the directions for regular granola. After the dehydration step, stir in ½ cup dried pineapple, ½ cup dried mango, and ½ cup dried coconut flakes.

Choco Granola

Follow the directions for regular granola. After the dehydration step, stir in ¼ cup cacao powder and ¼ cup carob powder. If you like, you can also add some cacao nibs for more crunch and flavor.

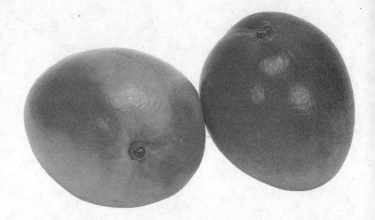

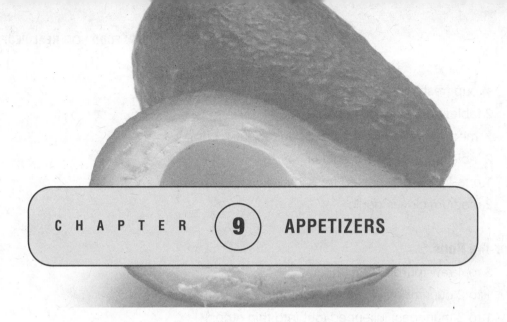

CHAPTER 9 APPETIZERS

Appetizers offer an opportunity to tickle the palate and stimulate the appetite. Raw-food appetizers are wide-ranging, from dishes as simple as a plate of sliced heirloom tomatoes and coconut drizzled with olive oil and sprinkled with oregano and sea salt to more complicated things such as pine-nut-pâté-stuffed rawvioli with a nutty mushroom sauce. With appetizers, we don't want to overwhelm the palate with overpowering flavors — think subtle and sublime.

NORI ROLLS WITH ATLANTIS PÂTÉ

These make a beautiful and elegant appetizer and are not as difficult to make as you might think. The trick is in rolling them. Other types of pâtés work well, too, so feel free to experiment. Be sure to use purple, not green, nori sheets, as the green ones have been toasted.

Makes 3 or 4 rolls (6 pieces per roll)

For the Atlantis Pâté
1 cup ground walnuts
1 carrot, finely grated (about ½ cup) (or use pulp left over from juicing carrots)

¾ cup fresh dill

2 tablespoons lemon juice

½ medium yellow onion, chopped (about ¼ cup)

2 tablespoons dulse granules

1 one-inch piece peeled fresh ginger

2 medium cloves garlic

For the Rolls

3 to 4 raw (purple) nori sheets

1 to 2 cucumbers, julienned (cut into thin strips)

1 to 2 mangoes, julienned (cut into thin strips)

1 to 2 avocados, julienned (cut into thin strips)

1½ to 2 cups alfalfa sprouts (see chart, page 57)

For the Shoyu Wasabi Sauce

6 tablespoons nama shoyu (substitute 1 tablespoon miso paste and
     6 tablespoons water to make gluten free)

1 teaspoon wasabi powder

Sunflower sprouts, alfalfa sprouts, and/or sprouted mung beans for garnishing
     (optional)

1. To make the pâté: Place all the pâté ingredients in a food processor and blend well until smooth.

2. Lay one nori sheet down on a board. Spoon about ½ cup pâté onto the sheet and spread evenly over one-third of the sheet. Place some cucumber, mango, and avocado strips on top of the pâté. Top with alfalfa sprouts, and roll, baby, roll. Seal the edge with a swipe of water. Repeat with the remaining ingredients.

3. To make the Shoyu Wasabi Sauce: In a small bowl, mix together the nama shoyu and wasabi powder until well blended.

4. Cut each roll into 6 to 8 slices. Place on plates and serve each with its own small ramekin of the Shoyu Wasabi Sauce. Garnish with sprouts, if you like.

MISO DULSE DIP

This recipe took me minutes to create after years of thinking about it. I have long been dipping celery into miso, but it's really too strong and salty. Finally one day I mixed together some miso with Cashew Kreme Cheeze and created this incredibly yummy dip! It's delicious with vegetable crudités.

Makes 3 cups

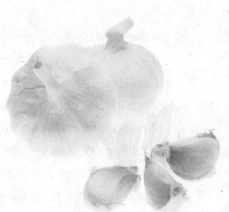

1 medium lemon, peeled and quartered

¾ cup mild miso paste

1 teaspoon dulse granules

1 medium clove garlic

Dash of cayenne pepper

1 teaspoon peeled chopped fresh ginger

1 tablespoon coconut oil

½ cup water, plus additional (up to ½ cup) as needed

½ cup soaked cashews (soaked 2 hours, drained, and rinsed; you may want to soak a few more to have on hand to improve consistency of dip)

1. Put the lemon in a blender, then add the miso paste, dulse granules, garlic, cayenne, ginger, coconut oil, and ½ cup water. Blend well. Slowly add the cashews while blending, occasionally stopping to move the mixture with a spatula. If the mix gets too thick to blend more cashews into, add more water a teaspoon at a time and continue to add cashews. If the final mix is too thin (that is, more like a dressing than a dip), blend in more cashews until it has a thick dip consistency. Keep in mind, however, that once the mix cools in the fridge it will get significantly thicker.

2. Remove to a small bowl, cover, chill for one hour, and serve.

HEIRLOOM TOMATOES WITH COCONUT MOZZARAWLA

This makes a spectacular appetizer but it's really, really easy to make. Don't tell anyone it's not really mozzarella and see if they can tell the difference.

Serves 4

4 medium heirloom tomatoes
3 medium fresh coconuts
Cold-pressed olive oil for drizzling
2 teaspoons chopped fresh oregano for sprinkling
2 teaspoons chopped fresh basil for sprinkling
1 tablespoon sea salt for sprinkling
Juice of 1 lemon for drizzling
Basil leaves for garnishing

1. Cut the tomatoes crosswise into ⅓-inch-thick slices, and cut into halves.
2. Drain the coconut water from the coconuts and reserve for use in other recipes. Remove the coconut meat from the coconuts in large pieces (see instructions, page 51).
3. Cut the coconut into round pieces 1 to 2 inches in diameter.
4. Arrange the tomato pieces and coconut rounds on four plates. Drizzle with olive oil, and sprinkle with herbs and salt. Squeeze a little lemon juice (about 1 teaspoon) over each plate. Garnish with a few basil leaves and serve.

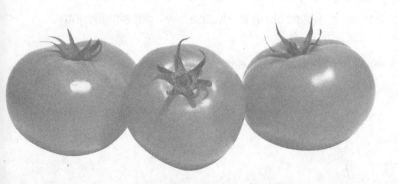

CASHEW KREME CHEEZE

I invented this spread one night after people had been asking me to make some for years. I don't know what took me so long, but it was worth the wait. This stuff is "bomb"! You can serve it with virtually anything edible — crackers, crudités, whatever — and it will taste great.

Makes 3 cups

1 medium lemon, peeled and quartered
1 tablespoon coconut oil
1 tablespoon agave nectar
Dash of cayenne pepper
1 tablespoon chopped fresh dill
1 medium clove garlic
2 teaspoons chopped yellow onion
1 teaspoon sea salt
½ cup water, plus additional (up to ½ cup) as needed
2 cups soaked cashews (soaked 2 hours, drained, and rinsed; you may want to soak a few more to have on hand to improve consistency of dip)

1. Put the lemon in a blender, then add the coconut oil, agave nectar, cayenne, dill, garlic, onion, salt, and ½ cup water. Blend well. Slowly add the cashews while blending, occasionally stopping to move the mixture with a spatula. If the mix gets too thick to blend more cashews into, add more water a teaspoon at a time and continue to add cashews. If the final mix is too thin (that is, more like a dressing than a dip), blend in more cashews until it has a thick dip consistency. Keep in mind, however, that once the mix cools in the fridge it will get significantly thicker.
2. Remove to a small bowl, cover, and chill for one hour.

VARIATIONS

Onion and Chive Cashew Kreme Cheeze

Follow the directions for regular Cashew Kreme Cheeze, but after removing to a bowl, mix in 1 tablespoon chopped yellow or spring onion and 1 tablespoon snipped fresh chives. Garnish with a sprig of chives and serve with crackers or crudités.

Kreme Cheeze and Lox

Follow the directions for Onion and Chive Cashew Kreme Cheeze and refrigerate. In a blender, combine ¼ cup dulse flakes with 1 tablespoon miso paste and ½ cup water and blend. Put ½ cup sun-dried tomatoes in a medium bowl and pour the dulse mixture over them; let marinate for 1 hour. Drain the tomatoes, cut them into strips, and mix them into the Kreme Cheeze. Garnish with strips of the marinated sun-dried tomatoes and serve on a piece of raw bread, or with crackers or crudités.

Mango and Coconut Cashew Kreme Cheeze

Follow the directions for regular Cashew Kreme Cheeze, but increase the amount of coconut oil to 3 tablespoons and the amount of agave nectar to 2 tablespoons. After removing to a bowl, mix in 2 tablespoons chopped fresh mango and 1 tablespoon dried coconut. Garnish with coconut flakes and mango slices and serve with crackers or crudités.

Cashew Kreme Cheeze Sliders

These delicious little sandwiches make great hors d'oeuvres. Prepare Cashew Kreme Cheeze and Artisan Herb Bread (see recipe, pages 74–75). Slather each slice of bread with a generous layer of Kreme Cheeze, then add a slice of tomato, some mesclun greens, and thinly sliced red onions, if you like.

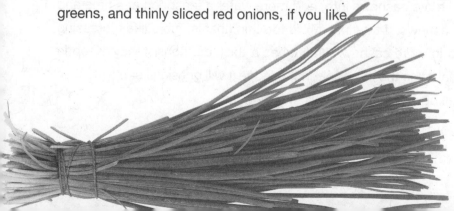

BABA GANOUSH

This is one of my favorite dishes from the Middle East, so I had to come up with a raw version. This is great with crudités or spread on crackers or bread. (Actually it's great by the spoonful as well!)

Makes 6 to 8 cups

2 large eggplants

1 teaspoon sea salt

2 cups sprouted sunflower seeds (see chart, page 59)

2 cups sprouted lentils (see chart, page 58)

½ cup nama shoyu (substitute ⅓ cup miso paste to make gluten free)

¾ cup cold-pressed olive oil

2 medium lemons, peeled and quartered

1 bunch fresh parsley leaves (about 1 cup)

½ teaspoon ground cumin

5 medium cloves garlic

1 tablespoon agave nectar

1 tablespoon sea salt

1 cup tahini

1. Roughly chop the eggplants and put them in a large bowl. Sprinkle with salt, cover with water, and let soak for 30 minutes.

2. Drain the eggplant and transfer it to a food processor. Grind thoroughly, and remove to a bowl.

3. Set aside a couple of parsley sprigs for garnishing. Then add the parsley and the rest of the ingredients except the tahini to the food processor and blend well. Add in the tahini and blend again. Remove to the bowl with the ground eggplant and mix well. Garnish with sprigs of parsley.

ONION RINGS

This is a raw version of a classic recipe. The onions are normally fried in oil, so we are going to trade the carcinogens for some extra flavor! The amaranth should be sprouted according to the chart on page 57, dehydrated until quite dry, and then ground into a powder in a food processor.

Serves 4

1 medium lemon, peeled and quartered
¾ cup cold-pressed olive oil
1 teaspoon curry powder
1 teaspoon nutritional yeast
1 teaspoon sea salt
2 large yellow onions
½ cup sprouted, dried, and ground amaranth (see chart, page 57)

1. Put the lemon, olive oil, curry powder, yeast, and salt in a blender and blend well.
2. Cut the onions crosswise into slices and separate into rings. Dehydrate the onion rings in a dehydrator for about 30 minutes.
3. Put the onion rings in a large bowl, pour the sauce over them, and marinate for about 10 minutes.
4. Dredge the onion rings in the amaranth powder and place on a dehydrator tray. Put the tray in the dehydrator and dehydrate the coated onion rings for 4 to 6 hours or until the coating is dry and slightly crispy. Serve while still warm. You will be amazed!

RAWVIOLI WITH MUSHROOM SAUCE

These are incredibly elegant served as an appetizer. They look like true homemade ravioli, taste pretty close to the cooked item, and are a delectable little treat.

Serves 4 to 6

For the Filling
½ pound cremini or portobello mushrooms, roughly chopped (about 1 cup)

¼ cup mild miso paste

¼ cup lemon juice

2 medium cloves garlic

½ bunch fresh parsley leaves (about ½ cup)

1 cup soaked pine nuts (soaked 2 hours and drained)

1 cup soaked macadamia nuts (soaked 2 hours, drained, and rinsed)

For the Wraps
4 large turnips or rutabagas

For the Mushroom Sauce
1 cup soaked cashews (soaked 2 hours, drained, and rinsed)

1 cup soaked almonds (soaked 8 to 10 hours, drained, and rinsed)

1 pound cremini or portobello mushrooms, roughly chopped (about 2 cups)

⅓ cup nama shoyu (substitute ¼ cup mild miso paste to make gluten free)

2 medium cloves garlic

4 cups warm water

4 parsley sprigs for garnishing

1. To make the filling: Put all the ingredients except the pine nuts and macadamias in a blender and blend well. Slowly add the nuts while blending, occasionally stopping to scrape down the sides of the blender jar with a spatula; add as many

nuts as possible while maintaining a smooth texture. Remove the filling to a bowl and chill.

2. Slice the turnips or rutabagas very thinly with a mandoline or slicer. The slices must be paper thin for this dish to really work because they act as the "pasta" in this version of ravioli.

3. Lay half the turnip or rutabaga slices out on dehydrator trays. With a spoon, drop about 1 teaspoon of filling onto each slice. Cover each one with another veg-etable slice and press the edges down so it looks like a little ravioli. Repeat until all slices and filling are used.

4. Put the trays in a dehydrator for about 30 minutes, just till the rawvioli are warm.

5. To make the Mushroom Sauce: When the rawvioli are almost done, put all the sauce ingredients in a blender and blend well.

6. Arrange the rawvioli on plates and spoon warm mushroom sauce over the top. Garnish with a sprig of parsley and serve immediately.

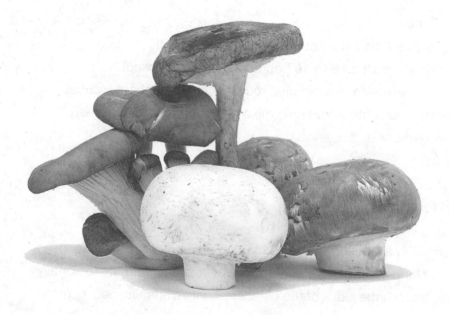

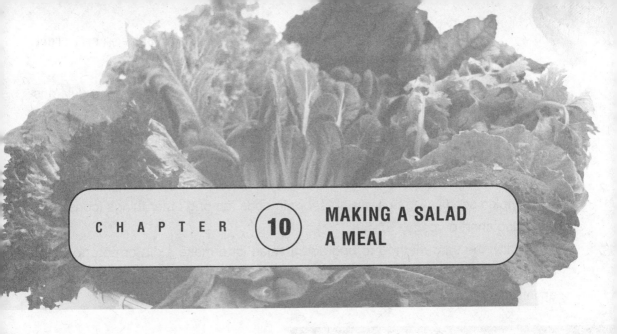

Okay, you've had a wonderful morning eating a nutritious and delicious breakfast. It's getting on toward lunchtime and you want to prepare a super salad. But you want something more than a simple salad of greens. How to turn a simple salad into an amazing meal? Please read on.

First of all, you might like to know that green leafy vegetables are in my opinion the most important foods for human beings to eat — in fact, they make life possible on the planet. Yep. Most people know greens are full of vitamins and minerals, but did you know that green leafy vegetables are actually good sources of protein? From where did you think cows get their protein? It ain't meat or dairy!

So how can we take our salads up a notch? I'm going to offer you a few ideas. The first is to take advantage of the great variety of greens available. There are so many delicious greens to choose from. Only a decade or so ago it seemed that iceberg was the only lettuce variety anyone ate in the United States. Now we have added spring mix and romaine, which are both delicious and good for you. And there are so many more types of lettuces and greens: dandelion is one of my favorites, as are the many varieties of kale, chard, bok choy, and so on.

The second method for improving your salads is simply to sprout some seeds or nuts and toss them on top. For instance, take some raw sunflower seeds and soak them in water for 6 to 8 hours. Then let them sprout in a jar or bucket for a day (rinsing them a couple of times). They will start growing a little tail and become soft and sweet. Rinse them again and put them in a closed container in the fridge. Then, any time you are making a salad, you can include a handful of fresh sprouts. This will add texture, nutrition, and yummy taste to your salad! Wow, what a gourmet! You can also try pumpkin seeds, wild rice, walnuts, or almonds, among other things (consult the sprouting chart on pages 57–59).

Finally, the third method to upgrade a salad is to make a dip or pâté to dollop over the top. Some of my favorites for this are hummus and guacamole, but there are an infinite number of possibilities.

SPROUTED CHICKPEA HUMMUS

Okay, I'm going to give it up here — my prized recipe for hummus. It's so easy, and it keeps well for a few days in the fridge. Besides being a great dip/appetizer, it also can turn any salad into a real meal. So make enough for a few days, and you'll always have a delicious and very nutritious boost to add to salads or wraps. Also, note that Tahini Sauce is a versatile ingredient you'll be able to use for many other recipes, so you're adding another dressing and dip to your raw repertoire as well! To use it as salad dressing, you can thin it with a little water.

Makes 6 cups

6 cups sprouted chickpeas (see chart, page 57)

For the Tahini Sauce
2 medium lemons, peeled and quartered
1 cup tahini
1 medium yellow onion, peeled and quartered
3 medium cloves garlic
½ cup fresh parsley leaves
½ cup fresh cilantro leaves

1 teaspoon ground cumin

⅓ cup cold-pressed olive oil

1 teaspoon sea salt, plus additional (up to 1 teaspoon) to taste

1. Put the sprouted chickpeas in a food processor and blend well. Remove to a large bowl.
2. To make the Tahini Sauce: Put the lemon first, then the remaining ingredients, in a blender and blend well.
3. Pour the Tahini Sauce into the bowl with the chickpeas and mix well. Taste and adjust the seasonings. Voilà!

VARIATIONS

Sprouted Chickpea Hummus with Sun-Dried Tomatoes

Follow the directions for Sprouted Chickpea Hummus, but add ⅓ cup sun-dried tomatoes to the ingredients in the blender. Blend well, then cut another ⅓ cup sun-dried tomatoes into thin strips and stir them into the hummus. This way, you get the wonderful flavor of these tomatoes throughout the hummus as well as getting delicious concentrations of their flavor and a nice chewy texture.

Sprouted Chickpea Hummus with Black Olives and Chives

Follow the directions for Sprouted Chickpea Hummus, but add ⅓ cup chopped sun-dried or oil-cured black olives (available online and in some specialty stores) to the ingredients in the blender. Blend well, then stir another ⅔ cup of the olives plus ½ cup chopped chives into the hummus. Again, you get wonderful flavor mixed through the hummus as well as delicious concentrations of flavor and a differentiated texture.

The process we just followed to make hummus can be repeated with different ingredients to make a huge variety of dips, pâtés, breads, and so on. You grind up a base, make a sauce, and then mix them together.

Don't believe me? Okay, let's make one right now! Okay, what do I have? That is always the first question I ask when I am going to make something. I look all around, inside the fridge and in the cupboards, and make a sort of inventory in my head of what I have. And then an idea forms — step-by-step — as I begin seeing what I want to do with it next. I don't often have the whole plan in mind. Usually it's a general concept and more a feeling, and then it gets more and more in focus until it is just right, sharp and clear. Go ahead, try it yourself. What do you have on hand? What do you want to use up? What do you feel like eating? Now you probably already have some ideas forming. What will be the base? What do you have to make a sauce that will work with your base? Experiment with proportions, taste it as you go along, smell it, check the consistency, and add your favorite ingredients. Enlist your creativity! And have fun.

Guacamole is another perennial favorite salad booster — although the truth is that everything tastes good with guacamole and almost everybody likes it! Many people, however, have never even tasted real guacamole. Real guacamole is not the homogeneous green goo with a two-month shelf life that's sold in many supermarkets. Guacamole is a very simple dip but can have a complexity of texture and taste.

To me, the secret of an outstanding guacamole is the avocado. Sound a little obvious? Well, you see, guacamole is often blended in a food processor, which creates an evenly smooth green spread that may taste good but has no variety of texture and frankly might be made from just about anything with a green hue.

What I love is the avocado, so I want chunks of avocado in my guacamole! Seeing and tasting real chunks of avocado lets me know this is the real thing. One way to achieve the desired consistency is to slice your avocados in half and remove the pits, take a spoon and scoop out each half avocado in one piece, and then put them on your cutting board and chop them up with a chef's knife. This way you can choose the size of the pieces and even have a variety of sizes.

When making a larger quantity of guacamole, I found a great tool for chopping up the avocados. I was getting really tired of chopping up a hundred of them at a time with a knife, and I started thinking about how to make it go faster. First I tried a potato masher. The result was some chunks with lots of goo — you see, the masher was actually squishing the avocado rather than slicing it. So I thought some more, and from somewhere out of my subconscious, the memory of my dad teaching me to make apple pies when I was a kid popped into my head. (Don't worry — later on I'm going to teach you how to make a really delicious and satisfying raw apple pie that even my dad loves.)

To make pie crust, one cuts shortening into a flour mixture with a special tool called a pastry blender. This is a D-shaped item with a handle and curved blades or wires that are about a quarter of an inch apart. You can find these in most kitchen supply stores. The purpose of this tool is to combine the fat and flour while keeping the dough as light and airy as possible. The blades actually cut through the dough instead of mashing it.

Guess what? It works perfectly for guacamole! Armed with a pastry blender, you can chop a big bowl of avocado halves into the exact size chunks you want in minutes. And the pastry blender doesn't mash; it slices — that's the key!

By the way, if you don't have a pastry blender, you can use a fork or two. Try holding two forks together side by side and using them to mash your avocados. They will mash more than they slice, but they still work pretty well. And let's face it, it's pretty hard to mess up guacamole!

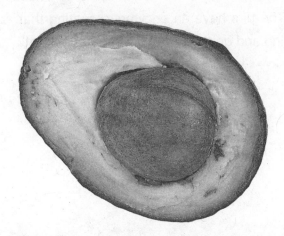

HOLY MOLY GUACAMOLE

This is a delicious, chunky guacamole that people will remember. If you like, you can mix in chopped tomatoes, mangoes, bell or chili peppers, or anything else your creative impulses lead you to add!

Makes 5 to 6 cups

8 medium avocados
1 medium lemon, peeled and quartered
½ medium yellow onion, roughly chopped (about ¼ cup)
3 medium garlic cloves
2 tablespoons cold-pressed olive oil
½ bunch fresh cilantro leaves (about ½ cup)
1 tablespoon sea salt, or to taste

1. Cut the avocados in half lengthwise and remove the pits. With a spoon, scoop out each avocado half in one piece. Using a pastry blender, chop the avocado into whatever size pieces you prefer. Put in a large bowl.
2. Put the lemon in a blender, add the rest of the ingredients, and blend well. Add this sauce to the chopped avocados, and gently mix.

A final tip on guacamole: If you are going to store it for any length of time, add the pits back in, cover, and refrigerate. The pits have an enzymatic coating that actually inhibits the avocados from oxidizing and going brown! Isn't nature brilliant?

Now I am going to teach you how to make my favorite day-to-day salad. It's a salad and dressing all in one, and all you need to make it is a bowl and a knife! This recipe was taught to me by my daughter's mom, Jeannette Rotondi, an excellent chef.

Kale is one of my favorite foods. There are many varieties — green curly kale, black kale, dinosaur kale, and many others. Let's use the most readily available one, green curly kale, to make this recipe.

Often kale is used on salad bars as a garnish but is not eaten. Because it is so curly, it might seem almost indigestible at first. We are going to use that curliness to trap and hold on to dressing and flavors. Here's the recipe.

HALE KALE SALAD

This is the basic recipe for a delicious and quick kale salad. You can of course add other ingredients (unless you want them to be mashed in, add them after you have completed the basic recipe). Some of my favorite additions are sprouted wild rice, tomatoes, seaweed, mung bean sprouts, and tahini. Yummy — I'm getting hungry just thinking about them!

Serves 1 to 2

1 bunch kale leaves
1 medium avocado
Juice of 1 medium lemon (about ½ cup)
Dash of cayenne pepper
½ teaspoon sea salt

1. To prepare the kale leaves: Holding a kale leaf by the stem with one hand, wrap your other hand around the leaf up near the stem with your thumbnail exerting a slight pressure on the stem. Glide your thumbnail down the stem, separating the leaf from the stem; once you get the technique, it's a snap. Using this technique, deleaf one bunch of kale leaves into a large bowl.

2. Now, reach in and grab a handful of kale leaves and rip them into pieces. Continue this motion repeatedly until you have ripped all the leaves into small bite-sized pieces (you don't want the pieces to be too big because they could catch in the throat while you are swallowing or may just be unappetizing).

3. Cut the avocado in half lengthwise and remove the pit. With a spoon, scoop out each avocado half onto the kale leaves. Add the lemon juice, cayenne, and salt to taste.

4. Okay, now comes the fun part. Remember how I talked before about having a relationship with your food? Well, here is a chance to develop a very tactile and immediate bond! I want you to get down and dirty. Reach into that bowl and start mashing the mixture with your hands. Squeeze the avocado between your fingers. Mash it all up until you have all the kale bits coated in a lovely creamy sauce. (If no one is looking you might even go ahead and lick that tasty dressing off your hands when you're done.)

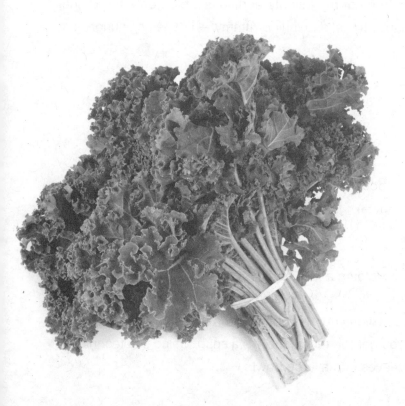

CAESAR IN THE RAW SALAD

The dressing for this salad is my personal favorite. It has just the right bite to it that makes me want more and more. For a thicker dressing, you can add more cashews. If you want to really go for it, sprinkle the salad with a teaspoon of spirulina and liberally shake on some more cayenne. You can also dress it up with red bell peppers and sprouted sunflower seeds.

Serves 4 to 6

2 heads romaine lettuce

For the Caesar Dressing

1 cup lemon juice

¼ cup miso paste

1 cup cold-pressed olive oil

4 medium cloves garlic

¼ cup apple cider vinegar

¼ teaspoon cayenne pepper

1 half-inch piece fresh ginger

Pinch of curry powder

3 tablespoons dulse flakes

2 cups soaked cashews (soaked 2 hours, drained, and rinsed)

1 to 2 cups Italian Croutons (see recipe, page 72)

¼ to ½ cup Rawmesan Cheeze (see recipe, pages 70–71)

Red bell peppers for garnishing (optional)

Sunflower seed sprouts for garnishing (optional)

1. Prepare the romaine by tearing off the outermost pieces and tossing them in your compost bin. Then cut off the stem end of the head and remove the leaves one

by one, rinsing them in water and tearing them into bite-sized pieces before putting them into a salad spinner or colander to dry.

2. To make the Caesar dressing: Combine all the ingredients in a blender and blend until smooth.

3. The final step is putting it all together. I sometimes drizzle the dressing over the salad without tossing it. A more traditional approach is to toss the whole salad with dressing, croutons, and Rawmesan. To follow this approach, pour enough dressing over the greens to coat them evenly but not so much that the salad gets soupy. Add most of the croutons and most of the Rawmesan Cheeze. Placé on a serving dish or platter. Sprinkle the rest of the Rawmesan Cheeze and the croutons over the top and garnish with bell peppers, sunflower seed sprouts, or anything else that suits your fancy. Mangia!

VARIATION

Caesar in the Raw Wrap

Carefully slice off the thickest part of the stem of a good-sized collard green, being careful not to cut the leaf. Place about 2 cups of Caesar salad along the spine of the collard green. Then just roll it up to make a really delicious wrap (see the instructions for the Bedouin Burrito on pages 118–19).

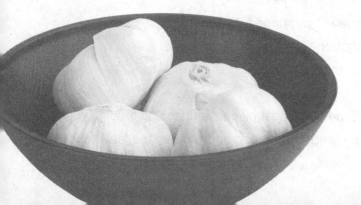

WAKAME WONDER SALAD

This is one of my favorite seaweed salads. Wakame is a wonderful sea vegetable —
easy to work with, delicious, and incredibly full of vital minerals.

Serves 4 to 6

6 cups dried wakame, broken into pieces
1 cup Leaf Organics House Dressing (see recipe, page 113)

1. In a large bowl, cover the wakame with water. Soak overnight. This removes much
   of the saltiness.
2. Rinse and drain the wakame well. Chop into 1-inch strips.
3. Toss the wakame strips with the house dressing, allow to marinate for 1 hour, and
   serve.

RAW SLAW

I often try to create raw substitutes for the foods I love. I always loved coleslaw, for
instance, but I wanted an optimally healthy option. This one came out perfectly. To
speed the preparation of the cabbages and carrots, you can use the slicing and grating attachments of your food processor.

Serves 6 to 8

½ medium head red cabbage, shredded or cut into very thin slices
   (about 2½ cups)
1 medium head green cabbage, shredded or cut into very thin slices
   (about 5 cups)
8 medium carrots, shredded (about 4 cups)

For the Dressing

¼ cup sprouted sunflower seeds (see chart, page 59)

3 tablespoons cold-pressed olive oil

¼ cup apple cider vinegar

¼ cup agave nectar

1 one-inch piece fresh ginger, peeled and chopped (about 1 tablespoon)

¾ cup water

1. Put the cabbages and carrots in a large bowl.
2. To make the dressing: Put all the ingredients in a blender and blend well.
3. Pour the dressing over the cabbage and carrots. Mix well, and you are ready to go!

POTATOLESS SALAD WITH LEMON DILL SAUCE

Bring this to your next barbecue, but don't tell your friends that it's raw and nutritious until after they have tasted it and swooned! As with many raw-food recipes, this involves simply chopping up a base, blending a sauce, and then mixing them together.

One of the main players in this recipe is jicama, which gives a crunchiness to the salad. If you prefer a less-crunchy salad, try using yellow squash instead of the jicama.

Please note that I don't recommend eating the skin of the jicama. To remove the skin, hold the jicama in your free hand solidly against your cutting board and slice off the skin piece by piece. It takes a bit of patience but works fine. Dicing jicama can be a little tricky because jicamas can be large and tough. For directions on slicing, dicing, and chopping, see chapter 5; follow my dicing instructions with extra care.

Serves 6 to 8

1 pound fresh jicama, diced (about 4 cups)

2 to 3 medium ribs celery, cut into ⅓-inch-thick slices on the diagonal
(about 1 cup)

1 large bell pepper (not green), diced (about 1 cup)

Kernels of 2 ears fresh corn (frozen can work in a pinch) (about 1 cup)

3 medium zucchini, diced (about 1 cup)

For the Lemon Dill Sauce

1 lemon, peeled and quartered

2 tablespoons agave nectar

2 tablespoons coarsely chopped fresh dill

½ teaspoon ground turmeric

½ cup soaked pine nuts (soaked 2 hours and drained)

½ cup soaked cashews (soaked 2 hours, drained, and rinsed)

½ to 1 cup water (add as needed)

1 teaspoon sea salt

1. Put the jicama, celery, bell pepper, corn, and zucchini in a large bowl.
2. To make the Lemon Dill Sauce: Put the lemon, agave nectar, dill, and turmeric in the blender and blend well. Then, while blending, slowly add the pine nuts and cashews and continue blending until smooth. Add water as needed.
3. Pour the Lemon Dill Sauce over the veggie mix and stir well.

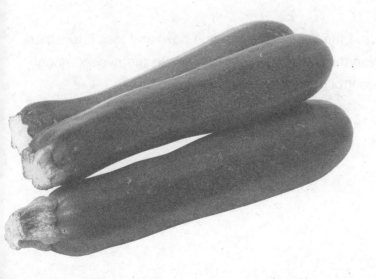

WILD RICE PILAF

Though sprouting wild rice might sound like a chore, it's really easy. However, you need to soak the rice for three days, so allow enough lead time. During the soaking process, the rice will swell, burst, and become soft, and it will end up with a wonderful nutty flavor. This makes a great side dish for dinner, an awesome filler in a wrap, or a delicious topping to a salad.

Serves 3 to 4

1½ cups sprouted wild rice (see chart, page 59)
1 tablespoon mild miso paste
3 tablespoons flaxseed oil
¼ cup lemon juice
2 teaspoons minced fresh oregano
¼ bunch fresh parsley leaves, minced (about ¼ cup)
1 to 3 large tomatoes, minced (about 2½ cups)
1 teaspoon ground cinnamon
½ teaspoon ground nutmeg
½ teaspoon sea salt
2 medium avocados, roughly chopped (about 1 cup)

1. Put all the ingredients except the avocados in a large bowl and toss it together using your hands until everything is mixed well. Then add the avocados and retoss; this way, you can control how much you mash them.

DRESSINGS

Keeping your salads interesting is one of the keys to a successful raw-food regime. However, drowning your salads in dressing in order to liven them up is kind of defeating the purpose. Dressings are an accent, not the main theme. Let the dressing interplay with and bring out the flavors of the salad. If the dressing overwhelms the salad, its healthy balance has been lost.

With this in mind, I am going to teach you the basic recipe for our original House Dressing at Leaf Organics.

LEAF ORGANICS HOUSE DRESSING

This is a very tangy, gingery, creamy dressing that lights up your taste buds and wonderfully accentuates the taste of greens. You don't need much of it because it is so flavorful.

Makes 3 cups

1 lemon, peeled and quartered
½ cup nama shoyu
2 one-inch pieces peeled fresh ginger, chopped (about 3 tablespoons)
¾ cup cold-pressed olive oil
3 cloves garlic
¾ cup water

1. Put the lemon first, then all the rest of the ingredients except the water, in a blender. Blend well. Add the water and blend well again. Serve chilled. The dressing may be stored in the refrigerator for up to 2 weeks.

GLUTEN-FREE HOUSE DRESSING

The only ingredient I use in my restaurants that has gluten is nama shoyu, a raw soy sauce made with both wheat and soy. For those who wish to avoid gluten entirely, I recommend using sea salt, miso paste, seaweed, or celery juice to substitute for nama shoyu in your recipes. Here is a gluten-free and even creamier version of our house dressing.

Makes 6 cups

1 lemon, peeled and quartered
⅓ cup miso paste
2 tablespoons dulse flakes
2 one-inch pieces peeled fresh ginger, chopped (about 3 tablespoons)
¾ cup cold-pressed olive oil
3 cloves garlic
1 cup water

1. Put the lemons first, then all the rest of the ingredients except the water, in a blender. Blend well. Add the water and blend well again. Serve chilled. The dressing may be stored in the refrigerator for up to 2 weeks.

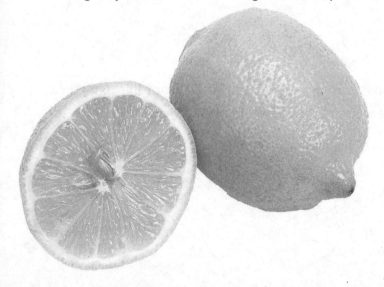

REALLY RAW RANCH DRESSING

Dressings and sauces are often what really set off a dish and get people excited. Try this raw ranch dressing — people love it!

Makes 5 cups

½ lemon, peeled and cut in half
1¼ cups soaked cashews (soaked 2 hours, drained, and rinsed)
½ cup soaked pine nuts (soaked 2 hours and drained)
¼ cup cold-pressed sesame oil
1 tablespoon agave nectar
¼ cup chopped fresh fennel bulb
½ teaspoon poultry seasoning
½ teaspoon chopped fresh dill
¾ cup apple cider vinegar
3 medium cloves garlic
1 teaspoon ground celery seed
1 cup water
¼ cup cold-pressed olive oil

1. Put the lemon first, then all the rest of the ingredients, in a blender. Blend well. Serve chilled. The dressing may be stored in the refrigerator for up to 2 weeks.

POMEGRANATE DRESSING

This is one of my favorite dressings, especially with dandelion greens or arugula. The sweetness of the dressing balances perfectly with the slight bitterness of the greens. Top the greens with pine nuts and pomegranate kernels, and you have an awesome salad.

Makes 3 to 4 cups

½ medium lemon, peeled and cut in half

1 half-inch piece peeled fresh ginger

½ cup fresh pomegranate kernels (properly known as "arils")

¾ teaspoon sea salt

½ cup cold-pressed olive oil

1 cup orange juice

1 cup soaked cashews (soaked 2 hours, drained, and rinsed)

2 tablespoons agave nectar

1. Put the lemon first, then all the rest of the ingredients, in a blender. Blend well. Serve chilled. The dressing may be stored in the refrigerator for up to 2 weeks.

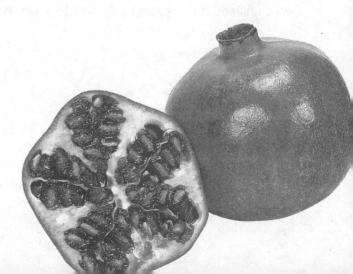

A NOTE ABOUT OILS

As a side note, I would like to mention that there are some schools of thought in the raw-food movement that eschew the use of any oils. Most notable in this regard is an approach known as "natural hygiene." Proponents of this practice believe that any food that is not a whole food is not optimal for human consumption. Thus an oil, which is separated from the whole food from which it is made, is not good.

I have never tried this approach because it has never appealed to me from an intellectual, intuitive, or culinary standpoint. Nevertheless, I am happy to pass this on to any of you who might find it interesting.

Just keep in mind that it is never some abstract idea that matters. Make your food choices because something works for you, not because you like the idea of it. If you like an idea, try it out, then listen to your body. The more you listen, the more you will be able to hear what it is saying to you. Body awareness is like a muscle — if you don't use it, it atrophies. If you exercise it daily, it will get stronger and stronger.

WRAPS

Another way to keep your salads interesting, change up the texture, and make them seem more substantial is to turn them into wraps. For years I worked on coming up with the best wrapper to make wraps. I tried dehydrating combinations of sprouted grains, greens, and many other ingredients. Then one day at a farmers' market, my eyes fixed on some collard greens and I had a revelation. Of course! Nature had already invented the perfect wrappers — I didn't need to do it. Collard greens work beautifully as wrappers, as do many other leafy greens. In fact, they have been using grape leaves in the Middle East for exactly this purpose for thousands of years. So let's get this wrapped up.

BEDOUIN BURRITO

Of course, the same process you use to make this wrap can be re-created with any kind of pâté, croquette, or patty, or any combination of delicious raw, vegan, and organic ingredients you choose. Yummy!

Makes 1 wrap

1 collard green or other large edible leaf
½ cup mixed greens
½ medium tomato, cut into slices
2 tablespoons Leaf Organics House Dressing (optional, see recipe, page 113)
1 cup Sprouted Chickpea Hummus (see recipe, pages 100–101)
¼ cup Tahini Sauce (see recipe, pages 100–101)
6 to 8 sunflower sprouts
¼ cup alfalfa sprouts

1. Place the collard green leaf on a cutting board with the dark green side down. With a sharp knife, keeping the flat side of the blade almost parallel to the cutting board, slice away the center rib of the leaf from where it starts getting thick all the way to the end of the leaf where it is quite thick, keeping the leaf as intact as possible. The idea here is to remove as much of the thick rib as possible without cutting the leaf in half.
2. Add a bed of mixed greens along the stem line to cover where the rib was cut out.
3. Place 3 to 4 slices of tomato along the same line, leaving about 2 inches uncovered on either end.
4. Sprinkle the greens and tomatoes with the dressing, if using. Then scoop on the hummus and pour on the Tahini Sauce.
5. Lay the sunflower sprouts over the top, then cover everything with the alfalfa sprouts, so the sprouts act as a sort of blanket. This will allow you to close the wrap without too much mess.

6. Wrap it up! With two hands, lift the edge of the leaf closest to you up and partially over the filling. Keeping your right hand holding the folded portion, use the left hand to fold in that side's uncovered end of the leaf. Roll the wrap with both hands until the left end is securely tucked in. Then switch to the other side and do the same, finally rolling the wrap over the remaining edge of the leaf, forming the shape of a log. Cut in half on the diagonal, and serve on a plate.

Well, that should get you off to a good start with salads, dressings, and wraps. Use what you have learned here to branch off into your own creativity. Always tune in to what is available, fresh, and local. Remember, there is a huge variety of greens available if you know where to look. And growing your own greens, even microgreens in an apartment, is lots of fun.

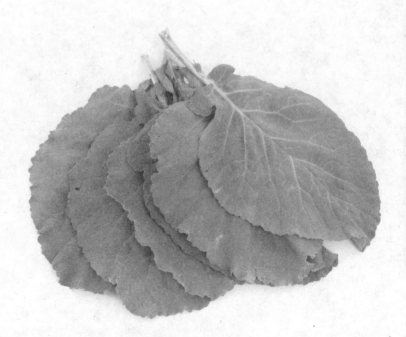

CHAPTER (11) SOUPS

Soups lend themselves extremely well to raw-food preparations. It's so easy to blend together some delicious ingredients, or even juice and then blend them. Keep in mind that most people associate soup with heat. There are some well-known cold soups, such as gazpacho or vichyssoise, but they are the exceptions.

There are two ways to heat a raw soup. You can heat it carefully on a burner on low heat, stirring constantly and either using a thermometer for temperature control (you don't want to exceed 110°F) or else testing it with a thumb or forefinger (when the soup starts to get uncomfortably hot to the touch, take it off the burner). Or you can make a soup with about half the liquid, and when you are ready to serve it, you simply add an equal amount of hot water, bringing the soup to the proper temperature and consistency. The recipes in this chapter use the second method.

Also, for each soup recipe, I have based the yield (for example, "Serves 6") on a serving size of one cup per person. If the soup will be a main course rather than a starter, or if you simply prefer larger servings, plan accordingly.

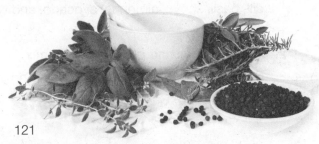

MIDDLE EASTERN LENTIL SOUP

I learned to love lentil soup when I lived in the Middle East. There they use a potent combination of tahini and cumin to flavor the soup. It is absolutely delicious, and the cumin is believed to help neutralize any gaseous effects the sprouted lentils might cause.

Serves 6

1 medium lemon, peeled and quartered
¼ cup cold-pressed olive oil
4 cups sprouted lentils (see chart, page 58)
1 one-inch piece peeled fresh ginger, chopped (about 1 tablespoon)
1 medium clove garlic
1 teaspoon ground cumin
⅛ teaspoon cayenne pepper
1 tablespoon sea salt
¼ cup fresh dill
4 basil leaves
¼ cup nama shoyu (substitute an extra teaspoon of sea salt to make gluten free)
½ cup soaked almonds (soaked 8 to 10 hours, drained, and rinsed)
½ medium avocado
1½ cups water
¼ cup tahini
Hot water for heating
Chopped parsley for garnishing

1. Put the lemon first, then the olive oil, lentils, ginger, garlic, cumin, cayenne, salt, dill, basil, shoyu, almonds, avocado, and water, in a food processor. Process until smooth.
2. Add the tahini and process just to mix.
3. Before serving, heat the soup by stirring in very hot water in a 1 to 1 ratio of hot water to soup. Garnish with parsley.

MEXICAN CORN CHOWDER

This has become one of the favorite soups at our restaurants. It's easy to make at home — but please still come to the restaurants!

Serves 8

Kernels of 8 ears fresh corn (about 6 cups)
1 large yellow onion, chopped (about ¾ cup)
1 medium bell pepper (not green), chopped (about ½ cup)
1 to 2 medium cloves garlic
½ bunch fresh cilantro leaves (about ½ cup), plus more for garnishing
¾ cup lemon juice
1 teaspoon ground cumin
Dash of cayenne pepper
Sea salt to taste
Hot water for heating

1. Set aside ½ cup corn kernels for garnishing. Put the remaining corn kernels and all the other ingredients except the hot water in a blender. Blend until smooth with some chunky bits, adding water as needed. If you like it chunkier, lightly blend the mixture, then remove a third of it to a small bowl. Blend the remaining two-thirds until smooth, then add in the chunky portion and blend just to mix.
2. Before serving, heat the soup by stirring in very hot water in a 1 to 1 ratio of hot water to soup. Garnish with extra corn kernels and cilantro.

VARIATION

Kids' Corn Chowder

To make a milder version for kids, leave out the onion, garlic, and cayenne. My daughter, Lilli, can't get enough of it. She often requests it for breakfast!

KREME OF BUTTERNUT SQUASH SOUP

This is a perfect creamy fall soup — earthy and flavored with spices to warm you from the inside. You can also easily add in more curry or cayenne to create a spicier soup.

Serves 8

1 medium lemon, peeled and quartered
2 cups water
½ cup soaked sunflower seeds (soaked 2 hours, drained, and rinsed)
1 medium clove garlic
1 half-inch piece peeled fresh ginger
¼ teaspoon curry powder
¼ teaspoon cayenne pepper
½ teaspoon sea salt
3 pounds butternut squash, peeled, seeded, and chopped (about 3 cups)
2 medium carrots, chopped (about 1 cup)
¼ cup tahini
Hot water for heating
Chopped parsley for garnishing

1. Put the lemon first, then the 2 cups water, sunflower seeds, garlic, ginger, curry powder, cayenne, and salt, in a blender. Blend until smooth. Add the squash and carrots and blend again.
2. Add tahini and blend again just to mix.
3. Before serving, heat the soup by stirring in very hot water in a 1 to 1 ratio of hot water to soup. Garnish with parsley.

KREME OF ASPARAGUS SOUP

This is a creamy, slightly Asian take on a classic. You could even substitute broccoli or cauliflower for the asparagus to change it up.

Serves 4 to 6

2 cups soaked cashews (soaked 2 hours, drained, and rinsed)
2 cups soaked Brazil nuts (soaked 2 hours, drained, and rinsed)
1 cup water
½ cup miso paste
1⅓ pounds fresh asparagus, chopped (about 4 cups)
1 medium clove garlic
Hot water for heating
Chopped parsley for garnishing

1. Put the cashews, Brazil nuts, and 1 cup water in a blender and blend until the liquid is smooth and silky.
2. Add the miso, asparagus, and garlic and blend again.
3. Before serving, heat the soup by stirring in very hot water in a 1 to 1 ratio of hot water to soup; the soup should be thick and creamy. Garnish with parsley.

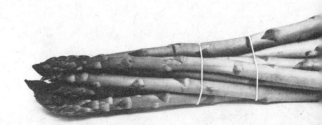

KREME OF MUSHROOM SOUP

This beats that canned soup any day! Oh yeah, and it's not loaded with salt and dairy products. People can't believe how easy and delicious this soup is.

Serves 8 to 10

½ cup soaked cashews or macadamia nuts (soaked 2 hours, drained, and rinsed)
2 cups soaked almonds (soaked 8 to 10 hours, drained, and rinsed)
3 cups water
⅔ cup nama shoyu (substitute tamari or ½ cup miso paste to make gluten free)
2 pounds fresh button mushrooms, chopped (about 4 cups), plus extra for
    garnishing
2 medium cloves garlic
Hot water for heating

1. Put the nuts and 3 cups water in a blender and blend until the liquid is smooth and silky.
2. Add the nama shoyu, mushrooms, and garlic and blend again.
3. Before serving, heat the soup by stirring in very hot water in a 1 to 1 ratio of hot water to soup; the soup should be thick and creamy. Garnish with chopped mushrooms.

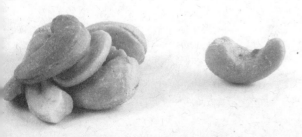

SPANISH GAZPACHO

I find this to be a wonderfully refreshing and tasty soup! The little bit of apple cider vinegar really brings out the tastes in a lovely way. An ideal summer soup, gazpacho is traditionally served raw and cooled.

Serves 5 to 6

¼ cup cold-pressed olive oil

6 medium fresh tomatoes, roughly chopped (about 6 cups)

1 medium onion, chopped (about ½ cup)

1 large bell pepper (not green), chopped (about ¾ cup)

1 medium clove garlic

1 small cucumber, chopped (about 1 cup)

4 basil leaves

1 tablespoon sea salt

1 large carrot, shredded (about ¾ cup)

¼ cup apple cider vinegar

Chopped fresh parsley and/or basil for garnishing

1. Combine all the ingredients in the bowl of a food processor, and process until blended but still chunky. Remove half of the soup to a large bowl and blend the remainder well. Pour the mixture from the food processor into the bowl and stir to blend.

2. Chill for 1 hour; garnish with parsley and/or basil, and serve.

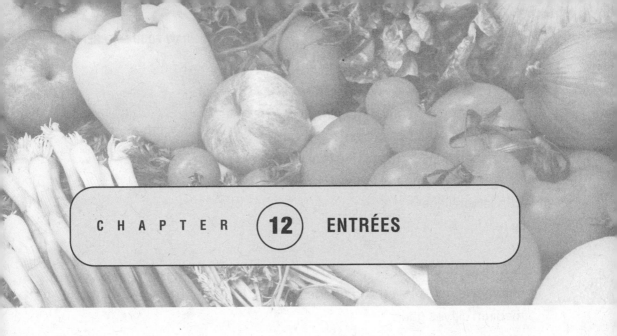

CHAPTER (12) ENTRÉES

Entreés are traditionally the most substantial part of the meal. The entrée is the main attraction, so it's an opportunity to really show your stuff. We are going to learn some sophisticated entrées, such as Rawsagna, as well as some simpler ones, such as Pad Thai. Sophisticated or simple, they are all delicious and satisfying. And they also all provide well-balanced nutrition.

RAWSAGNA

Many people think of traditional lasagna as a difficult dish to make, but it's not really. It's just takes a little time to prepare the components in advance, and then you just layer them in a baking dish. This is a super easy and delicious raw version that will amaze your guests. If you use a mandoline to cut the squash, please be very careful not to cut yourself! Mandolines are notorious for being dangerous, and after all, we are trying to keep this a vegan dish!

Makes one 9-by-13-inch Rawsagna

For the "Pasta"

8 medium yellow summer squash

½ cup cold-pressed olive oil

1 teaspoon chopped fresh oregano

1 teaspoon chopped fresh basil

¼ cup lemon juice

Sea salt

For the Rawcotta Cheeze

1 medium lemon, peeled and quartered

3 medium cloves garlic

3 tablespoons chopped parsley

¼ medium yellow onion, chopped (about ⅛ cup)

3 tablespoons cold-pressed olive oil

1 teaspoon sea salt

½ cup water, plus extra for blending

½ cup soaked cashews (soaked 2 hours, drained, and rinsed)

½ cup soaked pine nuts (soaked 2 hours, drained, and rinsed)

2 cups Marinara Sauce (see recipe, pages 70–71)

½ cup Cheeze Sauce (see recipe, pages 70–71) and ½ cup Rawmesan Cheeze
    (see recipe, pages 70–71) for garnishing (optional)

1. To prepare the "pasta": Cut off the ends of the squash and use a mandoline or a
   sharp knife to cut it into long, flat slices about 1/16 to 1/8 inch thick. (A knife will work
   if you don't have a mandoline, but making thin, uniform slices with a knife is a
   challenge.) Pour the olive oil over these and sprinkle with oregano, basil, lemon
   juice, and a little sea salt, and toss well to coat. This will soften up the squash and
   give it a more pastalike texture.

2. To make the Rawcotta Cheeze: Put the lemon first, then the garlic, parsley, onion, olive oil, salt, and ½ cup water, in a blender and blend well. Slowly add the cashews and pine nuts while blending, adding water as needed, and continue blending until the mixture is the consistency of ricotta cheese.

3. To assemble the Rawsagna: Use a 9-by-13-inch lasagna pan that is not too deep. Cover the bottom of the pan with a layer of squash. Next, top the squash with a layer of Rawcotta, then add a layer of marinara on top of that. Repeat the layering until you run out of ingredients. The number of layers will depend on how thick you make each layer; I usually do 2 or 3 layers of each. Finish with marinara. Drizzle on the Cheeze Sauce and sprinkle on the Rawmesan Cheeze, if using. Place the pan in a dehydrator and dehydrate just enough to warm through (about 45 minutes), and serve. Delizioso!

VARIATIONS

Rawsagna with Extras

You can also feel free to add your favorite ingredients to the Rawsagna — fresh spinach, sun-dried tomatoes, and sun-dried olives are all delicious additions. You can add them on top as garnishes or create new layers — for instance, a layer of spinach between the squash and the Rawcotta.

Cannelloni

As an alternative, you can also use the same components to make cannelloni. Just take two squash slices and place them side by side, overlapping them slightly. Spread a dollop or two of Rawcotta on one end of the slices, and roll them up. Place seam-side down in a pan, and top with marinara. Place the pan in a dehydrator and dehydrate just enough to warm through (about 45 minutes), and serve.

PAD THAI

This staple Thai recipe is traditionally made with rice noodles and spicy peanut sauce, but there are many raw alternatives. Some stores sell kelp noodles that are organic and raw. I really like them, and they definitely satisfy the noodle hankering I get from time to time (the Pad Thai photo in this book shows the dish made with kelp noodles). But we are going to create our own version using thinly sliced coconut meat, mangoes, and bell peppers. People love this dish! Of course, you can also use these "noodles" with many different sauces, including the Marinara Sauce you learned when we made our Pizza Pizzazz (pages 70–71) and Rawsagna.

Serves 2

For the "Noodles"
2 medium mangoes, julienned (cut into thin strips)
1 medium bell pepper (not green), thinly sliced
Meat of 3 medium young coconuts, thinly sliced
½ teaspoon sea salt
Juice of 1 medium lemon (about ½ cup)
1 tablespoon cold-pressed olive oil

For the Spicy Nut Sauce
1 cup Nut Mylk (see recipe, page 78)
2 tablespoons nama shoyu (substitute tamari or 1 tablespoon miso paste to make gluten free)
¼ cup cold-pressed olive oil
¼ cup grated dry coconut
1 one-inch piece peeled fresh ginger
1 medium clove garlic
¼ cup chopped dates
½ bunch fresh cilantro leaves, chopped (about ½ cup)

½ teaspoon sea salt

¼ teaspoon cayenne pepper

Finely chopped walnuts for garnishing

Chopped fresh cilantro for garnishing

1. To make the "noodles": Put the mangoes, bell pepper, and sliced coconut in a large bowl. Add the salt, lemon juice, and olive oil, and toss to coat evenly. Allow to marinate for at least 20 minutes.

2. To make the Spicy Nut Sauce: Put all the ingredients in a blender and blend until smooth.

3. Pour any excess liquid off the "noodles." Pour the nut sauce over them and toss to coat. Top with chopped nuts and cilantro.

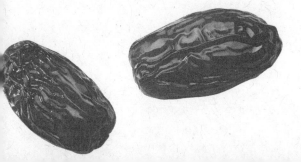

FISHLESS STICKS

This is a great comfort-food dish, wonderfully tasty and reminiscent of the deep-fried seafood sticks some of us grew up on.

Makes 12 to 14 sticks

For the Fishless Pâté
1 cup Brazil nuts, ground
½ cup sunflower seeds, ground
¼ cup sesame seeds, ground
2 tablespoons lemon juice
1 medium carrot, roughly chopped (about ½ cup)
1 small beet, roughly chopped (about ½ cup)
½ medium onion, chopped (about ¼ cup)
1 one-inch piece fresh peeled ginger
2 tablespoons dulse flakes
2 medium cloves garlic
¾ cup chopped fresh dill

For the Coating
½ cup sunflower seeds, ground
¼ cup sesame seeds, ground
¼ cup flaxseeds, ground
¼ teaspoon cayenne pepper
¼ teaspoon sea salt

For the Rawtar Sauce
1 medium lemon, peeled and quartered
¾ cup cold-pressed olive oil
¼ cup miso paste

1½ cups soaked cashews (soaked 2 hours, drained, and rinsed)

¼ medium yellow onion, minced (about ⅛ cup)

1 tablespoon minced fresh dill

1. To make the Fishless Pâté: Put the ground Brazil nuts, sunflower seeds, and sesame seeds in a large bowl. Put the remaining pâté ingredients in a food processor and process until smooth. Remove to the bowl with the Brazil nuts and sunflower and sesame seeds. Mix well by hand.

2. To make the coating: Put all the ingredients in a medium bowl and mix to combine.

3. Form the pâté into 3-inch-long fish-stick shapes, and roll them in the coating mixture to give them a breaded look.

4. Arrange the sticks on a dehydrator tray, put the tray into the dehydrator, and dehydrate for 8 to 12 hours or until the sticks are crispy on the outside and moist and yummy on the inside.

5. To make the Rawtar Sauce: Put the lemon, olive oil, and miso paste in a blender and blend well. Slowly add the cashews while blending, occasionally stopping to move the mixture with a spatula. Blend until smooth and creamy. Remove to a large bowl. Add the minced onions and dill. Mix to combine, chill for 1 hour, and serve.

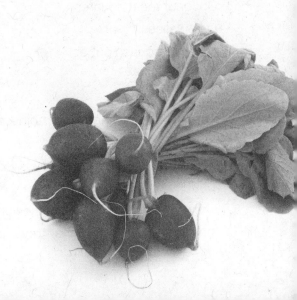

RAW VEGGIE SHISH KEBAB

This is a great dish for a barbecue or to serve a large group of people because it is so easy and people love it. You simply marinate veggies, skewer them, and then dehydrate them just long enough to warm and soften them up. We've suggested some of our favorite veggies, but you can use whichever are your favorites.

Makes 2 cups marinade, enough for about 10 to 12 skewers

For the Marinade
1 cup cold-pressed olive oil
⅓ cup nama shoyu (substitute ¼ cup miso paste to make gluten free)
½ cup water
1 medium clove garlic
1 one-inch piece fresh ginger, peeled and minced (about 1 tablespoon)
1 tablespoon poultry seasoning

Suggested Veggies
Bell pepper slices
Broccoli florets
Button mushrooms (whole)
Coconut meat squares
Onion slices
Summer squash cubes
Zucchini slices

1. To make the marinade: Combine all the ingredients in a blender and blend until smooth.
2. Put the veggies in a large bowl or pan and cover with the marinade. Marinate for 1 hour.
3. Skewer veggies with kebab skewers, alternating ingredients for visual variety. Put the skewers on dehydrator trays, put the trays in the dehydrator, and dehydrate

for 2 to 4 hours, periodically brushing on marinade. The kebabs are done when still moist but slightly wrinkled.

MEDITERRANEAN BURGERS WITH PESTO SAUCE

I originally created these in the form of croquettes at my first raw restaurant, Rod's Wrap & Juice Bar. Some of my customers dubbed these my "meatballs" because they have a very meaty consistency. The rich basil-infused pesto sauce creates a wonderful aroma and tastes divine. It also makes a great dressing or dip.

Makes 6 to 8 burgers

For the Patties

1 cup walnuts

1 cup hulled sunflower seeds

2 cups sprouted lentils (see chart, page 58)

½ cup coarsely chopped purple cabbage

1½ cups coarsely chopped celery (about 3 ribs)

1 medium lemon, peeled and quartered

1 cup sun-dried tomatoes, soaked 1 hour if not already soft

¼ cup cold-pressed olive oil

½ teaspoon sea salt

For the Pesto Sauce

1 medium lemon, peeled and quartered

1 cup spinach leaves

2 cups basil leaves

1 cup walnuts

1 cup cold-pressed olive oil

¼ cup garlic cloves (8 to 10 cloves)

½ bunch parsley leaves (about ¾ cup)

1 cup soaked cashews or pine nuts (soaked 2 hours, drained, and rinsed)

½ tablespoon sea salt

1 cup water, plus extra if needed

Romaine lettuce leaves, rinsed and dried

Red onion slices

Tomato slices

Alfalfa sprouts

1. Grind the walnuts and sunflower seeds in a food processor or coffee grinder. Remove to a large bowl.

2. Put all the other patty ingredients in a food processor and blend until the texture is fairly smooth but still has some small chunks.

3. Add the mixture from the food processor to the ground seeds and nuts and mix well. The mixture should then be a pâté-like consistency. If it's too wet, add some more grated sunflower seeds. If it's too dry, add some more water.

4. Use your hands to form the mixture into patties and place them onto a ParraFlex sheet on a dehydrator tray. Dehydrate 3 to 4 hours. Flip the burgers by inverting the dehydrator tray onto an empty tray without a ParraFlex sheet and then removing the ParraFlex sheet and the first tray.

5. Dehydrate for another 8 to 10 hours or until burgers are crispy on the outside but still a little spongy. These are best eaten warm right out of the dehydrator, but you can refrigerate them for up to a week if necessary.

6. To make the pesto sauce: Put the lemon first, then all the rest of the ingredients, in a blender. Blend well. (If you are using the pesto as a dressing, you might want it a little thinner; in that case, add more water to achieve the desired consistency.) Serve chilled. The pesto may be stored in the refrigerator for up to 2 weeks.

7. To construct your burger, place a leaf of romaine on your plate and set your patty on top of it. Spoon on 2 or 3 tablespoons of pesto sauce, then place a slice of red onion, a slice of tomato, and some alfalfa sprouts on top. Take another romaine leaf and cover the sandwich with it, wrapping the extra part of the leaf under the sandwich and around the back. Your burger is ready to go.

FLYING FALAFEL SANDWICH WITH COCO-CURRY SAUCE

Remember the Flying Falafel Croquettes from chapter 7? Well, here they are again, shaped like patties and served between two slices of mango bread. The lovely yellow sauce on this sandwich is one of my most popular sauces ever. It has a nice curry flavor with a coconut undertone and can also be used as a salad dressing or a dip. It's a winner! Of course, falafel is always good with Tahini Sauce (see recipe, pages 100–101), so you also could try this sandwich with that sauce.

Makes 4 sandwiches

For the Coco-Curry Sauce

1 medium lemon, peeled and quartered

½ cup cold-pressed olive oil

½ cup cold-pressed sesame oil

½ cup sprouted hulled sunflower seeds (see chart, page 58)

1 cup dried shredded coconut meat

½ cup soaked cashews (soaked 2 hours, drained, and rinsed)

⅓ cup agave nectar

1 two-inch piece fresh ginger

¼ cup garlic cloves (8 to 10 cloves)

½ teaspoon cayenne pepper

4 teaspoons curry powder

1 teaspoon sea salt

2 cups water, plus additional (up to 1 cup) as needed

4 Flying Falafel Croquette patties (see recipe, pages 66–67)

8 slices Mango Bread (see recipe, pages 73–74)

Red onion slices

Tomato slices

Alfalfa sprouts

Romaine lettuce leaves, rinsed and dried

1. To make the sauce: Put the lemon first, then the olive oil, sesame oil, sunflower seeds, coconut, cashews, agave nectar, ginger, garlic, cayenne, curry powder, salt, and 2 cups water, in a blender and blend well. (If you are using the sauce as a dressing, you might want it a little thinner; in that case, add more water to achieve the desired consistency.)

2. To assemble the sandwiches, place each falafel patty on top of a slice of bread. Spoon on 2 or 3 tablespoons of sauce, then add a slice of red onion, a slice of tomato, some alfalfa sprouts, and a romaine leaf or two. Top the sandwiches with another slice of bread, cut them in half, and serve.

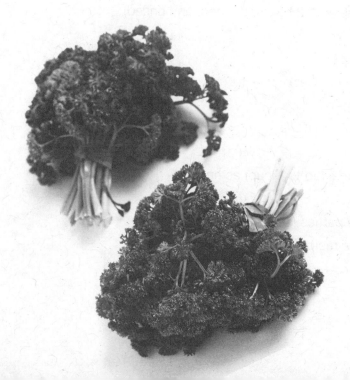

THANKSGIVING FEAST

Here are a few dishes to serve for a wonderful holiday meal. They are based around the traditional Thanksgiving meal, but with a raw vegan twist. We were running this as a special on Thanksgiving at the restaurant, and the Food Network came in and filmed me making it for a show called *The Secret Life of Thanksgiving*. It still airs every Thanksgiving. This meal is something to celebrate! If you like, you can choose a pie from the dessert chapter to complete the feast.

LOVE LOAF

If you are into making meat substitutes, then you should try this one. It is a very meaty and delicious dish. If you want to make it even more meaty, add a cup of soaked sun-dried tomatoes.

Makes 6 to 8 slices

½ cup sesame seeds, ground
⅓ cup flaxseeds, ground
¾ cup sunflower seeds, ground
Juice of 1 lemon (about ½ cup)
¼ cup mild miso paste
2 yams, chopped (about 2 cups)
1 medium yellow onion, chopped (about ½ cup)
1 medium apple, cored and chopped (about 1 cup)
8 sage leaves
1 small yellow summer squash, chopped (about ½ cup)
2½ teaspoons sea salt

1. Put the ground sesame seeds, flaxseeds, and sunflower seeds in a large bowl.
2. Put all the rest of the ingredients in a food processor and process until smooth. You can process this in batches if your machine can't do it all in one batch.

3. Add the processed vegetables to the ground seeds and mix together well.
4. Form the mixture into a long, low loaf, about 1½ inches thick, on a ParraFlex sheet. Put in the dehydrator and dehydrate for 10 to 12 hours, until the loaf is slightly crispy but still a little spongy.
5. To serve, cut the loaf into slices about ¾ inch thick and return them to the dehydrator for about an hour to warm and crisp up. Put a slice on each plate, and serve with Mashed Taters, Cranberry Sauce (recipes follow), and some greens.

CRANBERRY SAUCE

This sauce is simple but packs a lot of flavor. If you like, you can sweeten it even more with about ¼ cup agave nectar.

Serves 6 to 8

2 medium oranges, peeled and quartered
1 cup fresh cranberries (use frozen if you can't find fresh)
½ cup pitted dates
½ cup soaked walnuts (soaked 2 hours, drained, and rinsed)
1 medium yellow onion, chopped (about ½ cup)

1. Put the oranges first, then the rest of the ingredients, in a food processor. Process to your desired consistency. For a smoother sauce, you may remove some to a blender and blend until smooth, then return to the processor and pulse just to mix.

MASHED TATERS

This makes for a tasty and healthy comfort food. Smooth and delicious.

Serves 8

2 tablespoons lemon juice

2 cups soaked cashews (soaked 2 hours, drained, and rinsed)

2 small heads cauliflower, chopped (about 3 cups)

2 medium cloves garlic

2 teaspoons finely chopped rosemary

2 teaspoons sea salt

1. Put all the ingredients in a food processor. Process until smooth, about the consistency of mashed potatoes.

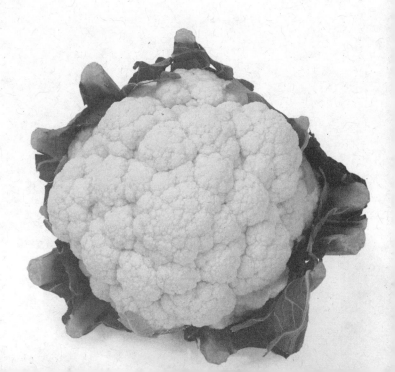

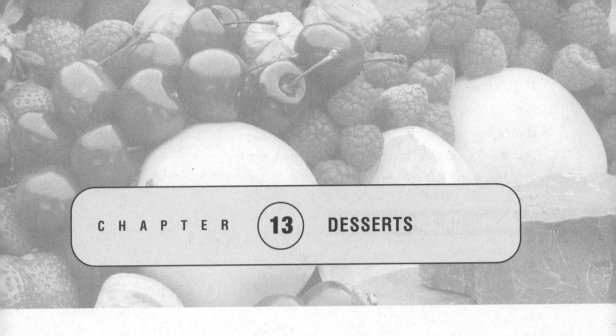

CHAPTER (13) DESSERTS

As good as any meal might be, it's the dessert that many people look forward to and often remember best! Happily, there are nearly infinite possibilities for raw desserts. In this chapter we will learn to make everything from brownies and mousse to pies and even ice kreme. And don't forget, dessert can be just some delicious seasonal fruits — it's hard to improve on mother nature (although a scoop of my Whipped Kreme might make that fruit even more delectable)!

LEMON ZINGER COOKIES

If you love the mixture of sweet and tart, then these cookies are for you. The lemon taste jumps out at you, and they're just sweet enough!

Makes 10 to 12 cookies

Juice of 1½ lemons (about ¾ cup)
1 cup soaked almonds (soaked 8 to 10 hours, drained, and rinsed)
¾ cup soaked dates (soaked 2 hours and drained)
1 tablespoon agave nectar

1. Put all the ingredients in a food processor and process until smooth.
2. Drop tablespoon-sized portions of the dough onto a ParraFlex sheet on a dehydrator tray and flatten them into cookie shapes.
3. Put the tray in the dehydrator and dehydrate the cookies for 4 to 6 hours, until slightly crispy but still moist.

BROWNIE BALLS OR BARS

Caution! Seriously addictive! These are sort of a cross between a Tootsie Roll and a traditional brownie.

Makes 24 balls or bars

2 cups chopped dates
½ cup carob powder
½ cup cacao powder
2 cups ground Brazil nuts
½ cup almond butter
½ cup grated fresh coconut for garnishing (may substitute dried)
Cacao nibs and/or goji berries for garnishing (optional)

1. Combine all the ingredients except the coconut and garnishes in a food processor and process until smooth.
2. Roll the dough into ¾-inch balls. Roll each ball in coconut, then in cacao nibs, if using, then press a goji berry into the top, if using. Place the balls on a baking sheet, and chill them for 2 hours. Alternatively, you can spread the dough about ⅓ inch thick on a baking sheet, sprinkle with dried coconut, and press in cacao nibs and/or goji berries, if using. Slice into bars and chill them for 2 hours. To extend the shelf life of the balls or bars, you can dehydrate them for 4 to 6 hours, until only slightly moist.

ROCKY ROAD BANANAS

Perfect for keeping in your freezer and pulling out whenever friends come over — or when you just get peckish! You can also use other nuts, such as pistachios, or add goji berries or other dried fruits.

Makes 6 bananas

1 cup Brazil nuts
1 cup walnuts
1 cup fresh coconut meat (may substitute dried)
½ cup raisins
6 bananas

1. Put the nuts, coconut, and raisins in a food processor and pulse until the mixture is blended but a little chunky.
2. Put the mixture in a shallow bowl or dish and roll the bananas in it. Set the bananas on a baking sheet, and freeze for at least 2 hours. Remove from the freezer 15 minutes before serving.

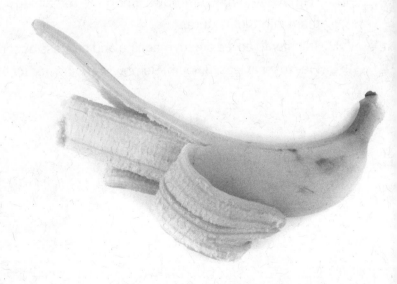

STRAWBERRY ICE KREME

Yes, it's true — raw ice cream is as good as or better than the dairy version. I challenge you to tell which is which! Many home ice cream makers work quite well. Most of them have a piece that needs to be well frozen before using. If you don't have an ice cream maker but you do have an extrusion juicer such as a Champion or Green Star, you can freeze the mix in an ice tray and then process the cubes through the juicer.

Serves 4

2 cups water
½ cup agave nectar
1 pint fresh strawberries, hulled (about 2½ cups)
¼ cup pitted dates
2 cups soaked cashews (soaked 2 hours, drained, and rinsed)

1. Put the water, the agave nectar, 2 cups of the strawberries, and the dates in a blender and blend. Slowly add the cashews while blending, occasionally stopping to move the mixture with a spatula. Blend until smooth.
2. Remove to a medium bowl. Chop the remaining ½ cup of strawberries and fold them into the mixture.
3. Transfer to an ice cream machine and process according to the instruction manual. Freeze for at least 3 hours. Remove from the freezer 10 to 15 minutes before serving.

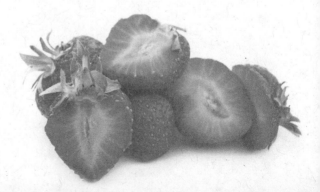

RASPBERRY VANILLA CHEEZECAKE

Here is a recipe from one of my colleagues at Leaf Organics, Noel Montenegro. He is a master with desserts. Thanks, Noel! As with all the recipes in this book, you can enlist your own creativity to come up with your own variations. We've included a recipe for a version with cacao below.

Makes 1 nine-inch cake

For the Crust

1 cup walnuts

½ cup Brazil nuts

½ cup almonds

½ cup chopped dates

1 tablespoon agave nectar

1 teaspoon ground cinnamon

Pinch of sea salt

For the Cheeze

⅓ cup agave nectar

⅓ to ½ cup water

Seeds from one vanilla bean, ground

2 cups soaked cashews (soaked 2 hours, drained, and rinsed)

For the Raspberry Sauce

1 pint fresh raspberries (about 2 cups)

½ cup agave nectar

1 teaspoon lemon juice

Pinch of sea salt

½ pint raspberries, chopped (about 1 cup), for garnishing

1. To make the crust: Put the walnuts, Brazil nuts, and almonds in a food processor and process until finely chopped. Add the dates, agave nectar, cinnamon, and salt and process until the mixture forms a ball.

2. Remove the dough to a 9-inch springform pan or pie pan and press the crust into the pan and up the sides with your hands, working to maintain an even thickness.

3. To make the Cashew Kreme Cheeze: Put the agave nectar, water, and vanilla seeds in a blender and blend well. Slowly add the cashews while blending, occasionally stopping to move the mixture with a spatula. Blend until smooth and thick.

4. To make the Raspberry Sauce: Put all the ingredients in a blender and blend until smooth.

5. To assemble the cake: Pour about a third of the Cashew Kreme Cheeze over the crust and spread evenly with the back of a spoon. Ladle about a quarter of the Raspberry Sauce onto the cheeze in a few blobs. Using a thin knife, swirl the blobs around to create a marbled look. Repeat to create a second level, and after you finish swirling, drop in most of the chopped raspberries. Finish with another layer of cheeze, then use the last of the Raspberry Sauce and the chopped raspberries to decorate as you wish.

6. Put in the freezer for at least 1 hour. Thaw for 15 minutes before serving.

VARIATION

Raspberry Cacao Cheezecake

Add ½ cup cacao powder to the Cashew Kreme Cheeze and add about ½ cup cacao nibs to the middle layer and some on top as a garnish.

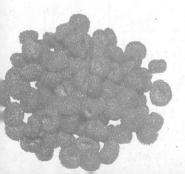

CUSHY CARROT CAKE

This is the healthiest carrot cake ever — and it's seriously delicious! The "frosting" can be eaten on its own. (And for that matter, so can the cake.)

Serves 8 to 10

For the Cake
6 medium carrots, chopped (about 3 cups), or 3 cups carrot pulp left over from juicing

1 cup soaked raisins (soaked 1 hour and drained)

2 cups coarsely chopped walnuts

½ teaspoon ground cinnamon

⅛ teaspoon ground cardamom

⅛ teaspoon ground nutmeg

¼ cup agave nectar

⅛ cup almond butter

For the Orange Cashew Kreme
½ cup orange juice

½ cup chopped pitted dates

1½ cups soaked cashews (soaked 2 hours, drained, and rinsed)

For the Orange Glaze
1 cup orange juice

1 tablespoon orange zest

1 tablespoon lemon zest

2 cups chopped pitted dates

1 tablespoon lemon juice

Dried coconut for sprinkling

1. To make the cake: If using chopped carrots, put them in a food processor and process to a pulp. Cut a large square of cheesecloth and line the bottom of a small bowl with it, letting the four corners hang over the edges of the bowl. Pour the pulp into the cheesecloth and then lift the four corners and twist them together. Lift the cheesecloth bundle and continue twisting the top to wring the liquid out of the pulp. Then put the dry pulp back into the food processor. (You may either drink the liquid in the bowl or discard it.) If using pulp left over from juicing, put it in the food processor. Then add the remaining cake ingredients and blend until the mixture reaches a doughlike consistency.

2. Remove the dough to a Parraflex sheet on a dehydrator tray and form it into a large rectangle about 1 inch thick. Dehydrate for 8 to 12 hours, until it reaches spongy, cakelike consistency. When you press it with your finger it should be a little soft and moist but not wet.

3. To make the Orange Cashew Kreme: Put the orange juice and dates in a blender and blend to combine. Slowly add in cashews while blending, occasionally stopping to move the mixture with a spatula. Blend until smooth, about the consistency of cake icing.

4. To make the Orange Glaze: Put all the ingredients in a blender and blend well.

5. To assemble the cake: Move the cake from the dehydrator tray to a serving plate or platter. Spread the Orange Cashew Kreme evenly over the cake. Drizzle with Orange Glaze, and sprinkle with dried coconut.

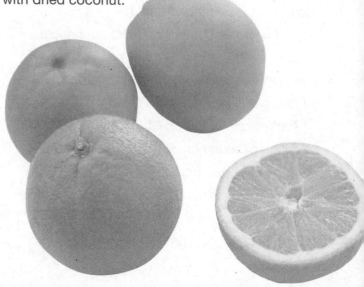

REALLY RAW APPLE PIE

Here is the raw recipe I modeled after my father's traditional apple pie. It's basically a date-nut crust filled with an apple compote, topped with Cashew Kreme and an apple-agave glaze. It's as beautiful an apple pie as you will ever see. And it's good for you!

Makes 1 nine-inch pie

Apple Compote and Glaze

6 medium Braeburn apples, cored and diced (about 6 cups)

¼ cup chopped soaked raisins (soaked 1 hour and drained)

2 tablespoons lemon juice

⅛ teaspoon ground nutmeg

⅛ teaspoon ground cinnamon

½ cup agave nectar

For the Crust

2 cups Brazil nuts

2 cups almonds

1½ cups chopped pitted dates

1 teaspoon ground cinnamon

½ teaspoon sea salt

For the Cashew Kreme

1 cup water

½ cup agave nectar

2 cups soaked cashews (soaked 2 hours, drained, and rinsed)

1. To make the Apple Compote: Put the apples in a large bowl. Add the raisins, lemon juice, nutmeg, and cinnamon and mix well. Let marinate for at least 1 hour.

2. To make the Apple Glaze: Put 2 cups of the Apple Compote in a blender. Add the agave nectar and blend well until smooth.

3. To make the crust: Put the nuts in a food processor and process until powdered. Add the dates, cinnamon, and salt and process until the mixture forms a ball. Remove to a deep-dish pie plate and mold it into a crust, using your fingers.

4. To make the Cashew Kreme: Put the water and agave nectar in a blender and blend to combine. Slowly add the cashews while blending, occasionally stopping to move the mixture with a spatula. Blend until smooth.

5. To assemble the pie: Scoop the compote into the crust until nearly full. Spoon the Cashew Kreme over the top, evenly covering the compote with a layer about ½ inch thick. Finally, drizzle with the apple glaze.

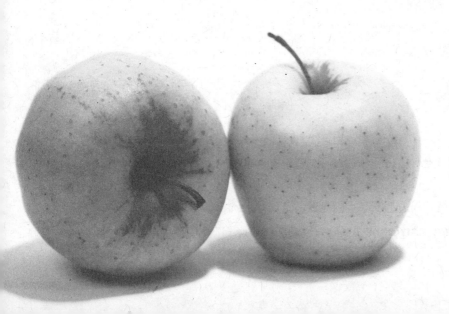

STRAWBERRY MOUSSE TARTLETS

This very elegant dessert has been one of our most popular desserts in our restaurants. You can also eat the mousse on its own!

Makes 8 to 10 tartlets

For the Strawberry Glaze and Mousse

½ pint fresh strawberries, hulled (about 1¼ cups)

1 teaspoon lemon juice

1 tablespoon agave nectar

1 teaspoon beet juice (optional; for color)

½ teaspoon sea salt

¾ cup soaked cashews (soaked 2 hours, drained, and rinsed)

For the Crust

1 cup Brazil nuts

1 cup almonds

1½ cups chopped pitted dates

1 tablespoon agave nectar

½ teaspoon sea salt

1. To make the Strawberry Glaze: Combine the strawberries, lemon juice, agave nectar, beet juice, and salt in a blender. Blend well. Remove half of the glaze to a bowl and refrigerate while making the mousse and crust.

2. To make the Strawberry Mousse: To the remaining glaze in the blender, slowly add the cashews while blending, occasionally stopping to move the mixture with a spatula. Blend until smooth and thick. Refrigerate while making the crust.

3. To make the crust: Put the nuts in a food processor and process until powdered. Add the dates, agave nectar, and salt and process until the mixture forms a ball. Divide the dough into little balls about 1½ inches in diameter, then form the balls into little tartlet shells, keeping the sides high and the center deep to hold as much mousse as possible.
4. Fill each tartlet with mousse, drizzle glaze over the top, and serve. Yummy!

CHOCOLATE BROWNIE SUNDAE

This is a wonderfully decadent chocolate treat made with real raw cacao, which the ancient Aztecs and Incans used to give to their warriors before battle. The amount of water in a coconut varies considerably, so buy three coconuts to be sure you get enough coconut water for the Whipped Kreme (you can drink any extra). You can also now buy coconut water in a carton, but I find that it tastes much better fresh!

Serves 12 to 14

For the Brownies

¼ cup agave nectar

¼ cup almond butter

5 medium carrots, finely grated (about 2½ cups)

¾ cup chopped soaked walnuts (soaked 2 hours and drained)

½ cup soaked raisins (soaked 2 hours and drained)

2½ cups raw cacao paste, nibs, or ground beans

¾ cup dried shredded coconut

⅛ teaspoon ground cinnamon

⅛ teaspoon ground nutmeg

¼ cup cacao powder

For the Whipped Kreme

1½ cups fresh coconut water (see note above)

½ cup agave nectar

6 cups soaked cashews (soaked 2 hours, drained, and rinsed)

For the Chocolate Sauce

1 cup agave nectar

2 tablespoons raw cacao powder

¼ cup soaked raisins (soaked 2 hours and drained)

Dried shredded coconut for garnishing

Chopped walnuts for garnishing

1. To make the brownies: Put all the ingredients in a food processor and process until fully smooth. Scoop onto a Parraflex sheet on a dehydrator tray and form into a large square, about ½ inch thick. Dehydrate for 10 to 12 hours, until it's slightly crisp on the outside but still spongy.
2. To make the Whipped Kreme: Put the coconut water and agave nectar in a blender and blend. Slowly add the cashews while blending, occasionally stopping to move the mixture with a spatula. Blend until as smooth and thick as possible. Refrigerate while making the sauce.
3. To make the Chocolate Sauce: Put all the ingredients in a blender and blend well.
4. To serve, move the warm brownies from the dehydrator tray to a serving plate or platter and cut them into squares. Cover them with Whipped Kreme in an even layer about ½ inch thick. Drizzle with Chocolate Sauce. Garnish with dried coconut and chopped walnuts, and serve.

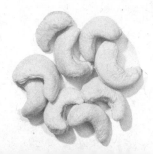

COCO CACAO MACA MOUSSE

This is a totally delicious mousse, which also gives you lots of energy. This will surely get any party going! Please note that the amount of meat in a coconut varies considerably, so buy five coconuts to be sure you'll end up with enough meat.

Serves 8 to 12

¾ cup agave nectar
2 cups fresh coconut meat (see note above)
½ cup maca powder
6 cups soaked cashews (soaked 2 hours, drained, and rinsed)
½ cup finely chopped cacao nibs

1. Put the agave nectar, coconut, and maca powder in a blender and blend well. Slowly add the cashews while blending, occasionally stopping to move the mixture with a spatula. Blend until as smooth and thick as possible.
2. Remove to a medium bowl, and mix in the cacao nibs.
3. Chill for at least 1 hour, and serve.

COCONUT MACAROON BALLS

These are a surefire crowd pleaser. The coconut coating gives them a gorgeous look, and the taste will keep people coming back for more.

Makes 10 to 12 balls

1 cup ground almonds (or you can use the pulp left over from making nut mylk)
1 cup chopped pitted dates, soaked 1 hour if not already soft
2 cups dried shredded coconut, divided

1. Combine the almonds, the dates, and 1 cup of the coconut in a food processor and process until the dough forms a ball.
2. Remove the dough from the food processor and form it into 1-inch balls. Roll each ball in the remaining coconut, place on a dehydrator rack, and dehydrate for 4 to 6 hours, until firm but not hard.

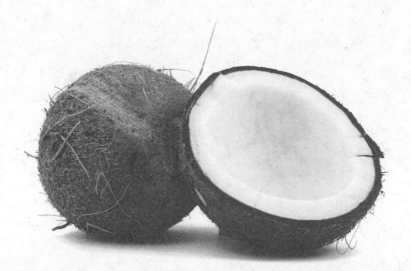

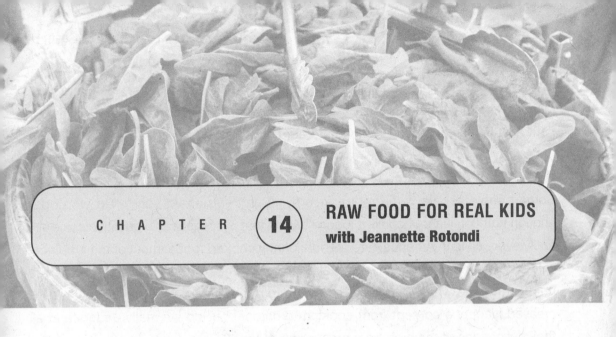

CHAPTER 14 RAW FOOD FOR REAL KIDS
with Jeannette Rotondi

I am very fortunate that my daughter's mom, Jeannette, practices a raw-food diet and is highly knowledgeable about many aspects of nutrition, health care, and holistic remedies. Because this is a large subject, we have written this chapter together, in order to share our combined experience and knowledge about raising kids raw.

Let's face it, anything to do with the health of our kids is a controversial and oftentimes contentious issue. So writing about a distinctly nonmainstream approach to nutrition for children is somewhat daunting. What we suggest here is that the vast majority of parents in this country are feeding their children a less-than-optimal diet that is at the root of many childhood ailments and ongoing health challenges.

Our three-year-old daughter, Lilli, is an incredibly healthy, happy, and physically strong and coordinated little girl. She has been eating a predominantly raw-food diet since birth. She loves seaweed for breakfast, guzzles green juice, will grab a handful of kale salad off someone else's plate and stuff it in her mouth with a big smile, and has never eaten refined sugar or flour in her life. She has never known the taste of sugary cereals, soda pop, French fries, meat, or dairy products. And she loves food. She even loves making food with us!

We feel great about feeding our child the uncompromised nourishment of a well-balanced organic living-foods diet comprising fruit, vegetables (including sea vegetables and fermented vegetables such as sauerkraut), sprouted grains, legumes, nuts, and seeds. Living foods are full of enzymes, balanced nutrients, water, and, yes, plenty of protein. What this really means is that we feed Lilli foods that are still in their natural state — unprocessed, unadulterated, and fresh.

IS RAW ENOUGH?

Some people ask us with great concern, "Aren't you afraid your child won't get enough nutrition without cooked foods?" While that is a reasonable question since virtually every child in America eats predominantly cooked foods, most of the empirical evidence even in the mainstream realm indicates that for the most part, food *loses* nutritional value when it is cooked. Yes, there are apparent exceptions, such as increased lycopene content from cooking tomatoes, but do we really understand all the implications of the high-heat processing of food?

We do know that digestive enzymes are destroyed by heat above 118°F. And if we back up and take a longer perspective on our eating habits, we note that every other animal on the planet, including other mammals, feeds its young raw foods. Needless to say, the benefits of having opposable thumbs and larger craniums, not to mention our Promethean leap, give us the choice of whether or not to cook our food, a choice other animals do not have. However, we might take note that animals in nature have an extremely low incidence of degenerative diseases, whereas those fed cooked foods suffer from a much higher incidence. We might also consider that humans ate raw foods for millions of years before the discovery of fire.

GROWING OUR KIDS

Now, we are not suggesting that starting tomorrow you eliminate all cooked foods from your child's diet. Rather, we are offering information and our experience, which might help you gradually adjust your children's relationship to food and the nutrition they get out of it. Nutrition is more than a prescription for recipes and meals. It is an opportunity for every parent to help forge for their kids a healthy and happy relationship with food. Example is often the best teacher, so a parent's own relationship with food is inevitably the most potent role model for our little ones. It might even be the best place to start.

Not so long ago, the majority of American families farmed, or at least having a garden in the backyard was common. Nowadays, that is the exception. It doesn't need to be. Cultivating a garden at home, or even just sprouting some simple things such as chickpeas or alfalfa seeds in the kitchen, will get your kids involved and interested in where food comes from. Even in the city, we can grow herbs in pots. Our daughter has fun watering plants and loves to nibble on sunflower greens. And let's face it — picking your own luscious little tomato is a special treat.

Making food with your children is fun, and it empowers them to have direct involvement in choosing and creating their foods. I know that with Lilli it's hard not to have her involved. She always has to be perched on a chair nearby so she can see everything I do. Recipes that involve actually getting your hands into the mix, such as our Hale Kale Salad (pages 105–6), are especially fun for little ones — they enjoy getting their hands messy and feeling the food.

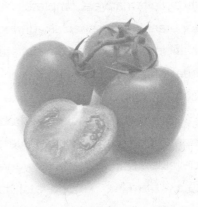

RAW BABY

So let's start at the beginning: infants. We are mammals, and breast milk is nature's finest, most complete baby food. Mother's milk is sweet, creamy, and easy to digest, containing simple sugars and free amino acids as well as plenty of good essential fatty acids, immune-supporting antibodies, and brain nutrients such as GLA and DHA. Its composition changes daily, responding to the unique needs of the developing child. No other food or man-made concoction can ever be as perfectly balanced and appropriate for an infant as its mother's milk. The World Health Organization recommends that children be exclusively breastfed during the first six months of their lives. One reason for this is that the lining of a child's intestines needs to mature. If solid foods are given before that process is complete, risks for allergies increase significantly.

Keep in mind that a mother's diet is critically important because it affects the quality of her breast milk and helps set the food preferences of the child. When the mother eats a well-balanced raw-food diet with correct supplementation, the milk is likely to be at optimal nutritional levels. To supplement a mother's diet, we recommend a DHA supplement that supports the healthy development of the child (as well as decreasing the possibility of postpartum depression). It is also essential for vegan nursing moms to supplement with vitamin B_{12} daily. Damages from B_{12} deficiencies are irreversible, so don't wait.

If breastfeeding is not possible, fresh goat's milk — not cow's milk — is the preferred alternative. Completely substituting plant-based alternatives such as nut mylk for breast milk, especially during infancy and before all the teeth have come in, is not sufficient, according to most studies. There is also evidence that soy milk, which is a heat-processed food, is not an optimal food for children because its high estrogen content may be unbalancing to the fragile hormonal system of a growing child.

Solid foods should be introduced gradually and according to the physical development of a child's digestive system (it takes approximately three years to fully develop). During the first two years of life, children need 50 percent of their caloric intake from fats — good fats! No wonder the perfect first solid foods to introduce are soft, tree-ripened sweet fruits such as bananas, and especially fatty fruits such as avocados and olives. An avocado is nature's perfect baby food. A little green vegetable juice diluted with water may also be given. Keep in mind that buying organic food ensures that your baby's diet will be free of pesticides, herbicides, genetically modified foods, and other highly questionable substances.

TODDLER EATS

If your child wants more variety but does not yet have all her teeth (especially the molars), you can expand her food choices considerably by prechewing complex carbohydrate foods such as greens or carrots. We recognize that many people will find this suggestion bizarre and irrational. A common, knee-jerk reaction is to assume that the practice is primitive and that only ignorant parents would prechew their children's food. But please consider that many animals in nature do this and, in fact, many other human cultures around the world do so as well. This method of food preparation for babies and toddlers has been practiced through the ages, and it provides them with nutrition far superior to what they would get from cooked foods.

Prechewing breaks down complex carbohydrates through digestive enzymes present in the mother's saliva. Infants do not manufacture these enzymes in sufficient quantities to break down these foods themselves. The emergence of a child's molars tends to coincide with the development of their enzyme production in sufficient quantity. If these complex carbohydrates are eaten frequently and not prechewed, they can impair proper development of the digestive tract. (Note, however, that prechewing food can transmit diseases, including HIV, strep, and hepatitis B.)

To prechew, take the normal amount into your mouth and chew it well, until it is completely masticated and wet. You can then mouth it onto a spoon to feed the child or you can feed mouth to mouth, as a mother bird feeds her young.

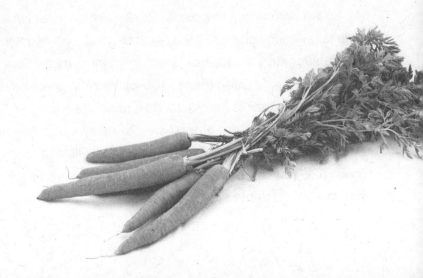

THE WELL-NOURISHED CHILD

After weaning, children (and teens and adults) can get sufficient nutrients, except vitamins B_{12} and D (when there is not enough exposure to sunlight), from a plant-based diet. However, it is wise to keep supplementing DHA. If your children have no allergy to flower pollen, it is highly recommended that you include this nutrient-dense food in their diets, because it not only provides protein that is easy to digest but also is an excellent source of lecithin, an important nutrient for the nervous system.

How much protein do kids actually need? The correct ratio is about 1 gram of protein per pound of body weight during the first year of life. This drops to about half a gram of protein per pound in the second through fifteenth years. If children eat enough calories from a balanced living-foods diet, they get plenty of protein. Excellent sources of protein include broccoli, leafy greens, chickpeas, lentils, nuts, and seeds. Soaking and sprouting the legumes, nuts, and seeds actually helps to predigest the nutrients and increases the amount of bioavailable proteins. The richest whole-food sources of protein are microalgaes such as spirulina and chlorella.

The reality is that most kids in this country are addicted to sugar, which is a major contributing factor in the epidemics of childhood obesity, diabetes, and ADD (attention deficit disorder). A recent study by Pennsylvania State University revealed that in the two- to three-year-old group, average consumption of added sugar was around fourteen teaspoons per day. This number jumped to seventeen daily teaspoons per day among four- and five-year-olds. Perhaps we can find other ways to reward our children than with processed sweets.

So we come back to greens. Green leafy vegetables are the key ingredient in an optimally healthy diet for kids as well as adults. Mixing and/or marinating greens and vegetables with avocados or dressings makes them more palatable. Kids of all ages love our Hale Kale Salad (pages 105–6). You can prechew or grind it for infants or toddlers, or serve it as is for older kids and adults.

Fruit smoothies are a great way to make quick food for kids. Chapter 8 offers recipes for lots of smoothies that your kids will love, such as the Virgin Piña Colada (page 82). You can even sneak some greens in, and they won't even know it. Add a handful of destemmed kale or spinach. You can also add goji berries, green powder, bee pollen, or chlorella for an extra nutritional boost. We recommend serving kids smoothies at room temperature or only slightly cooled. Cold food impairs digestion and is detrimental for children's developing gastrointestinal function.

Warmed raw soups with a moderate use of warming spices such as cardamom, cilantro, cinnamon, cumin, and ginger are especially beneficial for our youngsters. Kids' Corn Chowder (page 123) is one of Lilli's favorites.

I know that as my daughter grows up she will be exposed to many other food choices, and she might very well choose less-than-optimal foods. But at least I know that in her formative years, while it is still our choice, we are giving her the best foods nature has to offer.

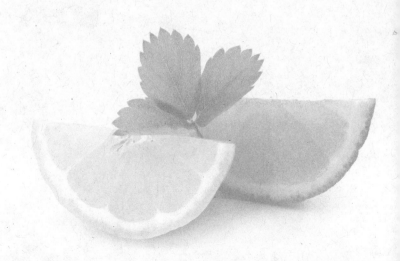

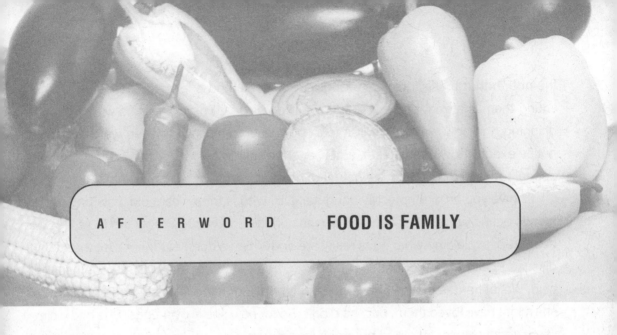

AFTERWORD   FOOD IS FAMILY

I grew up in an Italian American family, and food was often the thing that brought us together. No matter what daily issues came up, we all sat down to meals together. And holidays and weekends were often an opportunity for the extended family to gather and eat — and eat. Everyone would pitch in, so there was usually a crowd in the kitchen, all contributing to the feast. Dad would be making bread and pies, Mom would be making the main course and fixings, and the kids were enlisted as assistants — something we actually loved.

I know that many families no longer do this. That is a very fundamental change in both our relationship with food and how our families interact. Instead of lovingly crafting meals, many families now grab food out of a box or a microwave. My parents rarely resorted to these convenient yet compromised food sources. They wouldn't even let us eat "sugar cereals" — yep, severe deprivation.

Years later, I am grateful for their care and discernment. I think they gave us an important nutritional head start as well as a relatively healthy relationship with food. I say "relatively" because I have noticed that the foods we didn't get or got only on special occasions are the ones I have the strongest yearnings for.

I notice this with my little daughter — that if we withhold something from her, it almost inevitably becomes more interesting to her. So while we succeed in the short term in avoiding less-than-optimal foods for her, in the longer term we may be instilling the notion that these forbidden foods are special, and especially desirable — that eating them is a treat and a way to reward ourselves. For those of us with this conditioning, the only way to break it is to be present and aware when we eat, and to notice exactly how things taste, smell, and feel inside us. Most often a food's mythic appeal fades in the face of the actual thing.

I'll give you an example. My daughter, Lilli, who is three years old, saw one of her friends eating eggs at her house. Lilli was curious and wanted to try them. At first we demurred, explaining what eggs really are and why we don't eat them. But that didn't dissuade her. So we bought some organic, free-range eggs and made one with her help. We let her taste some, and she decided they don't really taste good at all. Sure, she might have loved them, but she didn't. So for now she is over eggs. She had a similar experience with steamed potatoes (her mom's side is German) — except she did like them and still does occasionally.

Another reason I say "food is family" is that many people use food to replace family and friends in their lives. No family or friends tonight? No problem. A pepperoni pizza and a pint of Ben and Jerry's, and that empty space inside will feel filled. It's what you might call medicating yourself with food, and it's a very widespread behavior.

Whom we eat with and what we eat are major determinants in who and what we are. And no matter how we grew up, we all have a choice as to what our next bite will be. You might not be able to choose your family, but you can choose your next meal and whom you'll share it with.

Some people have become scared of food. This is especially true in the raw-food movement. People are choosing their foods out of fear of other foods. I don't think this is healthy. I get customers sometimes who come in all uptight and worried about things, asking a million questions about very fine points. I think some of them don't really enjoy their food, which is a shame. Food is to be enjoyed! Whatever you choose to eat, enjoy it fully.

If you eat the healthiest foods in the world but do it out of fear, I truly believe that you will not gain the full nutritional benefits. And if you eat less-than-optimal foods, eat them with gusto and appreciation. Attitude and attention are powerful allies to conscious eating. Love your food, love your world, love yourself.

METRIC AND CELSIUS EQUIVALENTS

The equivalents below have been rounded for convenience.

Liquid and Dry Measures

U.S.	METRIC
⅛ teaspoon	.5 milliliter
¼ teaspoon	1 milliliters
½ teaspoon	2.5 milliliters
1 teaspoon	5 milliliters
1 tablespoon (3 teaspoons)	15 milliliters
¼ cup	59 milliliters
⅓ cup	79 milliliters
½ cup	118 milliliters
1 cup	237 milliliters
16 ounces	473 milliliters

Length Measures

U.S.	METRIC
¼ inch	6 millimeters
⅓ inch	8 millimeters
½ inch	1.27 centimeters
¾ inch	1.9 centimeters
1 inch	2.54 centimeters

Temperature

118°F = 47.78°C

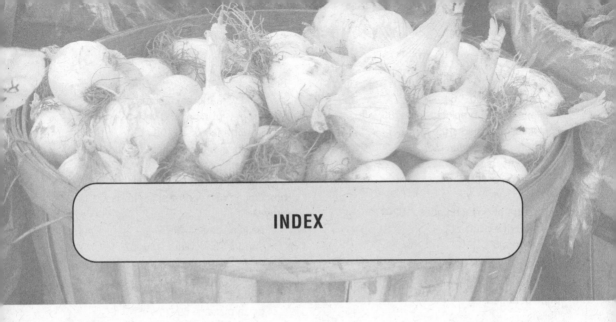

INDEX

A

acidity, 30–32
ADD (attention deficit disorder), 166
addictions, food, 21–22, 40–42
aging, premature, 27
alcohol, 32
alfalfa sprouts
    bedouin burrito, 118–19
    nori rolls, 90
alkalinity, 30–32
almond butter
    brownie balls or bars, 146
    chocolate brownie sundae, 156–57
    cushy carrot cake, 151–52
    real deal oatmeal, 83–84
almonds
    artisan herb bread, 74–75
    coconut macaroon balls, 159
    in dessert crusts, 149–50, 153–54, 155–56
    kreme of mushroom soup, 126
    lemon zinger cookies, 145–46
    Middle Eastern lentil soup, 122
    mushroom sauce, 97–98
    pizza pizzazz, 70–71
amaranth, in onion rings, 96

American Diabetes Association, 4
American diet. *See* SAD (standard American diet)
antibiotics, 30
antioxidants, 33
appetizers, 89
    baba ganoush, 95
    cashew kreme cheeze, and variations, 93–94
    heirloom tomatoes with coconut moz-
        zarawla, 92
    miso dulse dip, 91
    nori rolls with Atlantis pâté, 89–90
    onion rings, 96
    rawvioli with mushroom sauce, 97–98
    sprouted chickpea hummus, and variations,
        100–101
apple(s)
    love loaf, 141–42
    pie, really raw, 153–54
    real deal oatmeal, 83–84
    in smoothies, 81–82
artisan herb bread, 74–75
Ascended Health Products, 25
asparagus soup, kreme of, 125
Atlantis pâté, 89–90
attention deficit disorder (ADD), 166

avocados
    as baby food, 164
    buckwheat breakfast feast, 85
    hale kale salad, 105–6
    holy moly guacamole, 104
    Middle Eastern lentil soup, 122
    nori rolls, 90
    pits, 104
    preparation techniques, 102–3
    wild rice pilaf, 112
Ayurveda, 35

B

baba ganoush, 95
balls
    brownie, 146
    coconut macaroon, 159
bananas
    as baby food, 164
    keeping available, 48
    real deal oatmeal, 83–84
    rocky road, 147
    in smoothies, 81–82
bars, brownie, 146
basil, in pesto sauce, 137–38
bedouin burrito, 118–19
beets, in fishless sticks, 134–35
berry refreshing, 81
blenders, 45
blueberries, in smoothies, 81–82
blueberry bonanza, 81
body consciousness, 42
bowls, 46
Brazil nuts
    brownie balls or bars, 146
    in dessert crusts, 149–50, 153–54, 155–56
    fishless sticks, 134–35
    kreme of asparagus soup, 125
    nutter butter naner choco coco, 81
    rocky road bananas, 147
breads
    about, 73
    Italian herb, 72
    mango, 73–74

breakfast, 39–40
    buckwheat breakfast feast, 85
    groovy granola, and variations, 86–87
    importance of, 97–98
    real deal oatmeal, and variations, 83–84
    smoothies, 77–82
breastfeeding, 163–64
broccoli, in raw veggie shish kebab, 136–37
brownie
    balls or bars, 146
    sundae, chocolate, 156–57
buckwheat, sprouted
    artisan herb bread, 74–75
    breakfast feast, 85
    pizza pizzazz, 69–71
    porridge, living, 84
    protein dream, 82
burgers
    Mediterranean, with pesto sauce, 137–38
    veggie sun burger croquettes, 67–68
burrito, bedouin, 118–19

C

cabbage
    Mediterranean burgers with pesto sauce,
        137–38
    raw slaw, 109–10
    veggie sun burger croquettes, 67–68
cacao
    antioxidants in, 33, 80
    brownie balls or bars, 146
    choco granola, 87
    chocolate brownie sundae, 156–57
    coco cacao maca mousse, 158
    count choco maca oatmeal, 84
    raspberry cheezecake, 150
    in smoothies, 80, 81, 82
Caesar dressing, 107
Caesar in the raw salad, 107–8
Caesar in the raw wrap, 108
Cairney, Edward, 53
cake, cushy carrot, 151–52
California, 17–18
Camel Diving Safaris (Dahab, Egypt), 15

Campbell, T. Colin, 3
cancer, 4, 10, 22, 30
cannelloni, 131
Canyon Dive Club (Dahab, Egypt), 15
carob powder
    brownie balls or bars, 146
    choco granola, 87
    in smoothies, 81
carrot(s)
    artisan herb bread, 74–75
    Atlantis pâté, 89–90
    cake, cushy, 151–52
    chocolate brownie sundae, 156–57
    fishless sticks, 134–35
    flaxseed crackers, 64–65
    kreme of butternut squash soup, 124
    mango bread, 73–74
    pizza pizzazz, 69–71
    prechewing, 165
    raw slaw, 109–10
    Sicilian savory snaps, 65
    Spanish gazpacho, 127
    veggie sun burger croquettes, 67–68
cashew(s)
    Caesar dressing, 107
    coco cacao maca mousse, 158
    coco-curry sauce, 139–40
    kreme, 153–54
    kreme cheeze, 93–94
    kreme of asparagus soup, 125
    kreme of mushroom soup, 126
    lemon dill sauce, 111
    mashed taters, 143
    miso dulse dip, 91
    mushroom sauce, 97–98
    pesto sauce, 137–38
    raspberry vanilla cheezecake, 149–50
    rawcotta cheeze, 130–31
    rawtar sauce, 135
    really raw ranch dressing, 115
    strawberry ice kreme, 148
    strawberry mousse tartlets, 155–56
    whipped kreme, 157
cauliflower, in mashed taters, 143

celery
    Mediterranean burgers with pesto sauce,
        137–38
    potatoless salad with lemon dill sauce,
        110–11
    veggie sun burger croquettes, 67–68
cheeze
    cashew kreme, 93–94
    rawcotta, 130–31
    rawmesan, 70–71, 107
    sauce, 70–71
cheezecakes
    raspberry cacao, 150
    raspberry vanilla, 149–50
chickpeas, sprouted
    flying falafel croquettes, 66–67
    hummus, and variations, 100–101
children. See kids, raw food for
China Study, The (Campbell), 3
choco granola, 87
chocolate brownie sundae, 156–57
chocolate milk, 81
chocolate sauce, 157
chopping techniques, 49–50
chowder, Mexican corn, 123
cleansing, 42–43
Clement, Brian, 25, 26–27
Club Red Divers (Dahab, Egypt), 15, 16
coco cacao maca mousse, 158
coco-curry sauce, 139–40
coconut(s)
    chocolate brownie sundae, 156–57
    coco cacao maca mousse, 158
    coco-curry sauce, 139–40
    macaroon balls, 159
    and mango cashew kreme cheeze, 94
    mozzarawla, heirloom tomatoes with, 92
    mylk, 79–80
    opening, 51–52
    pad Thai, 132–33
    raw veggie shish kebab, 136–37
    rocky road bananas, 147
    tropical granola, 87
coconut water, 33, 51
coffee, 32

collard greens
    bedouin burrito, 118–19
    Caesar in the raw wrap, 108
    as wrappers, 117
compote, apple, 153–54
consciousness, 9, 42
cooked food
    disease resulting from, 22, 31–32, 36–37
    enzymes killed by, 28
    historical background of, 19–20
    nutrition lost through, 26–27
    oxygen lost through, 33
    pH imbalance in, 31–32
    raw food vs., 2
    transitioning from, 41–42
cookies
    brownie balls or bars, 146
    coconut macaroon balls, 159
    lemon zinger, 145–46
corn
    chowder, Mexican, 123
    cutting, 50
    potatoless salad with lemon dill sauce, 111
count choco maca oatmeal, 84
Cousens, Gabriel, 20, 25, 35–36
crackers
    about, 63
    flaxseed, 64–65
    Sicilian savory snaps, 65
cranberry sauce, 142
cravings, 22, 41
croquettes
    about, 66
    flying falafel, 66–67
    veggie sun burger, 67–68
croutons, Italian, 72
crusts
    for raspberry vanilla cheezecake, 149–50
    for really raw apple pie, 153–54
    for strawberry mousse tartlets, 155–56
cucumbers
    nori rolls, 90
    Spanish gazpacho, 127
cushy carrot cake, 151–52
cutting boards, 46

D
Dahab (Egypt), 14–16
dairy products, raw, 3
dates
    brownie balls or bars, 146
    coconut macaroon balls, 159
    cranberry sauce, 142
    cushy carrot cake, 151–52
    in dessert crusts, 149–50, 153–54, 155–56
    lemon zinger cookies, 145–46
    in smoothies, 81–82
    spicy nut sauce, 132–33
    strawberry ice kreme, 148
dehydration, low-temperature, 45
    breads, 73–75
    crackers, 63–65
    croquettes, 66–68
    general instructions, 62–63
    historical background of, 23–24
    pizza, 69–72
    process of, 61–62
dehydrators, 46, 61–63
desserts
    brownie balls or bars, 146
    chocolate brownie sundae, 156–57
    coco cacao maca mousse, 158
    coconut macaroon balls, 159
    cushy carrot cake, 151–52
    lemon zinger cookies, 145–46
    raspberry cacao cheezecake, 150
    raspberry vanilla cheezecake, 149–50
    really raw apple pie, 153–54
    rocky road bananas, 147
    strawberry ice kreme, 148
    strawberry mousse tartlets, 155–56
detoxing, 42–43
DHA, 164, 166
diabetes, 4, 10, 22, 30, 35–36, 166
dicing techniques, 50
dips
    baba ganoush, 95
    cashew kreme cheeze, and variations, 93–94
    coco-curry sauce, 139–40
    keeping available, 48

miso dulse, 91
pesto sauce, 137–38
sprouted chickpea hummus, and variations, 100–101
disease
degenerative, diet-based, 21, 22, 30
orthomolecularity and, 27
prechewing as cause of, 165
rates of, 10
raw alkaline diet and prevention of, 31–32, 35–36
vegetarian diets and reduction of, 3–4
See also specific disease
dressings. See salad dressings
dulse granules
Atlantis pâté, 90
Caesar dressing, 107
fishless sticks, 134–35
gluten-free house dressing, 114
miso dulse dip, 91

E
eggplants, in baba ganoush, 95
Egypt, 13–16, 61
Einstein, Albert, 4
electric ionic frequencies, 26–27
electrolytes, 33
electromagnetic energy, 34
emerald city oatmeal, 84
entrées
fishless sticks, 134–35
flying falafel sandwich with coco-curry sauce, 139–40
love loaf, 141–42
Mediterranean burgers with pesto sauce, 137–38
pad Thai, 132–33
rawsagna, and variations, 129–31
raw veggie shish kebab, 136–37
Enzyme Nutrition (Howell), 28
enzymes, 28, 61, 62
equipment, 45–46, 53, 103, 148
Essenes, 20

F
Fantasea Dive Club (Dahab, Egypt), 15
farmers' markets, 6
farming, 163
fasting, 42–43
fennel, in really raw ranch dressing, 115
Ferraro, Enzo, 16
fiber, 33–34
fishless sticks, 134–35
flaxseed
artisan herb bread, 74–75
crackers, 64–65
fishless sticks, 134–35
love loaf, 141–42
mango bread, 73–74
pizza pizzazz, 70–71
Sicilian savory snaps, 65
veggie sun burger croquettes, 67–68
flying falafel croquettes, 66–67
flying falafel sandwich with coco-curry sauce, 139–40
food, human relationship with, 4–7, 162–63
food addictions, 21–22, 40–42
food choices, 25
food contaminants, 3
food processors, 46
food security, 6
France, 12–13
fruit
buckwheat breakfast feast, 85
smoothies, 81–82, 166–67
See also specific type

G
Gandhi, Mohandas, 4
gardens, 4–5, 163
gazpacho, Spanish, 127
genetically modified organisms (GMOs), 3, 20
ginger
Atlantis pâté, 90
coco-curry sauce, 139–40
fishless sticks, 134–35
flaxseed crackers, 64–65
gluten-free house dressing, 114

ginger (*continued*)
  immuno blastoff, 81
  kreme of butternut squash soup, 124
  Leaf Organics house dressing, 113
  Middle Eastern lentil soup, 122
  pomegranate dressing, 116
  raw slaw, 110
  raw veggie shish kebab marinade, 136–37
  spicy nut sauce, 132–33
  veggie sun burger croquettes, 67–68
glazes
  apple, 153–54
  orange, 151–52
  strawberry, 155–56
gluten-free house dressing, 114
goat's milk, 164
grains, 32
granola, groovy, and variations, 86–87
greening, of sprouts, 54
green-juice fasting, 42
green lean scene, 81
greens
  bedouin burrito, 118–19
  prechewing, 165
  as protein source, 99
  as wrappers, 117
Greenwich Village (New York, NY), 9
guacamole
  holy moly, 104
  preparation techniques, 102–3
  as salad booster, 102
  storing, 104

H
hale kale salad, 105–6
health benefits of raw food, 2
  antioxidants, 33
  electromagnetic energy, 34
  enzymes, 28
  fiber, 33–34
  oxygen, 33
  pH balance, 30–32
  probiotics, 29–30
  research on, 25–27
  water, 33

health-food stores, 6
heart disease, 4, 10, 22, 30
heirloom tomatoes with coconut mozzarawla, 92
hemp protein powder, 80, 82
hepatitis B, 165
herb(s), 47
  bread, artisan, 74–75
  bread, Italian, 72
  gardens, 5
Hippocrates Health Institute (West Palm Beach, FL), 25, 27
HIV, 165
holy moly guacamole, 104
Howell, Edward, 28
hummus, 61
  as salad booster, 118–19
  sprouted chickpea, and variations, 100–101
hydration, 33
hygiene, natural, 117
hypertension, 4

I
ice cream makers, 148
ice kreme, strawberry, 148
immuno blastoff, 81
ingredients, 7
Italian croutons, 72, 107
Italian herb bread, 72
Italy, 11

J
jicama
  peeling, 110
  potatoless salad with lemon dill sauce, 110–11
juicers, 46
juices
  fasting with, 42, 43
  green vegetable, as baby food, 164

K
kale
  green lean scene, 81
  salad, hale, 105–6

kelp noodles, 132

kidney disease, 4

kids, raw food for

advantages of, 161–62

food relationships cultivated through, 162–63

infants, 163–64

nutritional concerns, 162

quick foods, 166–67

toddlers, prechewing for, 165

kids' corn chowder, 123

knives, 46, 49–50

kreme

of asparagus soup, 125

of butternut squash soup, 124

cashew, 153–54

of mushroom soup, 126

orange cashew, 151–52

whipped, 157

kreme cheeze

cashew, 93–94

and lox, 94

L

Leaf Cuisine (California restaurant chain), 17–18

Leaf Organics, 17, 18, 45, 54, 62

house dressing, 113

lecithin, 166

legumes, 47

lemon(s)

baba ganoush, 95

Caesar dressing, 107

cashew kreme cheeze, and variations, 93–94

coco-curry sauce, 139–40

-dill sauce, 111

fishless sticks, 134–35

gluten-free house dressing, 114

hale kale salad, 105–6

holy moly guacamole, 104

immuno blastoff, 81

kreme of butternut squash soup, 124

Leaf Organics house dressing, 113

love loaf, 141–42

mashed taters, 143

Mediterranean burgers with pesto sauce, 137–38

Middle Eastern lentil soup, 122

miso dulse dip, 91

onion rings, 96

orange glaze, 151–52

pad Thai, 132–33

pomegranate dressing, 116

preparing, 52

rawcotta cheeze, 130–31

rawtar sauce, 134–35

rawvioli with mushroom sauce, 97–98

really raw ranch dressing, 115

sprouted chickpea hummus, 100–101

tahini sauce, 100–101

zinger cookies, 145–46

lentils (sprouted)

artisan herb bread, 74–75

baba ganoush, 95

pizza pizzazz, 70–71

soup, Middle Eastern, 122

livestock industry, 4

Lord of the Rings trilogy (Tolkien), 73

love loaf, 141–42

lox, kreme cheeze and, 94

lunch, 40

M

macadamia nuts

cheeze sauce, 70–71

kreme of mushroom soup, 126

rawvioli with mushroom sauce, 97–98

macaroon balls, coconut, 159

maca root powder, 80, 81, 82, 84, 158

mandolines, 129

mango(es)

bread, 73–74

and coconut cashew kreme cheeze, 94

nori rolls, 90

pad Thai, 132–33

in smoothies, 81–82

tropical granola, 87

Marblehead (MA) Culinary Arts Festival, 12, 17

marinade, for raw veggie shish kebab, 136–37

marinara sauce, 70–71
mashed taters, 143
meat diet
    as acidifying, 30, 32
    fiber lacking in, 34
    historical background of, 19
    raw, 3
Mediterranean burgers with pesto sauce, 137–38
Mexican corn chowder, 123
Mexico, 11
Middle Eastern lentil soup, 122
miso
    Caesar dressing, 107
    dulse dip, 91
    gluten-free house dressing, 114
    kreme of asparagus soup, 125
    love loaf, 141–42
    rawtar sauce, 134–35
    rawvioli with mushroom sauce, 97–98
    wild rice pilaf, 112
mold, 48
Montenegro, Noel, 149
Morocco, 13
mousse
    coco cacao maca, 158
    strawberry, 155–56
mudslide slim, 81
mushroom(s)
    raw veggie shish kebab, 136–37
    sauce, 97–98
    soup, kreme of, 126
mylks
    coconut, 79–80
    nut, 78–79

N

natural hygiene, 117
Nature (magazine), 29–30
New York (NY), 9
"noodles," pad Thai, 132–33
nori rolls with Atlantis pâté, 89–90
nut(s), 47
    mylk, 78–79
    sauce, spicy, 132–33

    soaked, 48, 56
    See also specific type
nutter butter naner choco coco, 81

O

oat groat sprouts
    mango bread, 73–74
    real deal oatmeal, 83–84
    Sicilian savory snaps, 65
oatmeal, real deal, and variations, 83–84
obesity, 4, 10, 166
oils, 47, 117
olives
    as baby food, 164
    black, and chives, sprouted chickpea
        hummus with, 101
onion(s)
    and chive cashew kreme cheeze, 94
    raw veggie shish kebab, 136–37
    rings, 96
oranges/orange juice
    cashew kreme, 151–52
    cranberry sauce, 142
    glaze, 151–52
    green lean scene, 81
organic food, 3, 6
Organic Garden (Beverly, MA), 16
orthomolecularity, 27
oxygen, 33

P

pad Thai, 132–33
Palestine, 13–14
Palestinian cuisine, 13
pantry ingredients, 46–47
papaya, in smoothies, 82
Paris (France), 12–13
pastry blenders, 103
pâté
    Atlantis, 89–90
    fishless, 134–35
peppers
    pad Thai, 132–33
    potatoless salad with lemon dill sauce, 111

raw veggie shish kebab, 136–37
   Spanish gazpacho, 127
pesto sauce, Mediterranean burgers with, 137–38
pH balance, 30–32
pH Miracle, The (Young), 25
pie, really raw apple, 153–54
pilaf, wild rice, 112
pineapple
   in smoothies, 82
   tropical granola, 87
pine nuts
   cheeze sauce, 70–71
   lemon dill sauce, 111
   rawcotta cheeze, 130–31
   rawvioli with mushroom sauce, 97–98
   really raw ranch dressing, 115
pizza
   about, 69
   pizzazz, and variations, 69–72
   pizzazz abbondanza, 72
pollen, 166
pollution, 3, 4
pomegranate dressing, 116
porridges
   fruity oatmeal or buckwheat, 84
   living buckwheat, 84
   real deal oatmeal, 83–84
potatoless salad with lemon dill sauce, 110–11
prechewing, 165
pregnancy, 37
"Preventing and Healing Diabetes with a Raw-Food Diet" (Cousens), 35–36
probiotics, 29–30
"Probiotics: The Hidden Benefit of a Raw-Food Diet" (Rom Baba), 29–30
processed foods
   disease resulting from, 31–32, 36–37
   historical background of, 20
produce, 47
protein, 21–22
   children's needs, 166
   dream, 82
   greens as source of, 99
   hemp protein powder, 80

R

raisins
   chocolate brownie sundae, 156–57
   cushy carrot cake, 151–52
   real deal oatmeal, 83–84
   rocky road bananas, 147
ranch dressing, really raw, 115
raspberry/raspberries
   cacao cheezecake, 150
   and kreme, 82
   sauce, 149–50
   in smoothies, 81–82
   vanilla cheezecake, 149–50
"Raw Alkaline Diet, A" (Young), 31–32
raw-food diet
   adopting, 2
   as alkaline, 30
   author's discovery of, 9–10
   author's restaurants/businesses, 16–18
   exceptions to, 2
   as "extremist," 20
   flexibility of preparation, 7
   historical background of, 19–20
   human food relationships and, 4–7
   as lifestyle, 6–7
   as natural, 21
   organic food, 3
   preparation techniques, 7, 23–24, 45, 49–52
   simplicity of, 1–2
   vegan diet, 3–4
   See also health benefits of raw food; kids, raw food for; transitioning to raw-food diet
raw-food kitchen
   equipment, 45–46, 53
   pantry, 46–48
"Raw Foods: Your Body's Fuel" (Clement), 26–27
rawsagna, and variations, 129–31
rawtar sauce, 134–35
raw veggie shish kebab, 136–37
rawvioli with mushroom sauce, 97–98
Real Live Foods, Inc., 18
really raw apple pie, 153–54
really raw ranch dressing, 115

resourcefulness, as culinary skill, 11
restaurants, 10
Reversing Diabetes Naturally 21-Day Program, 35–36
Rishis, 20
rocky road bananas, 147
Rod's Wrap and Juice Bar (Marblehead, MA), 16–17, 137
Rom Bada, Compton, 25, 29–30
Rome (Italy), 11
Rotondi, Rod
    awards won by, 12, 17
    culinary education of, 10–13, 41, 61
    foreign diving businesses of, 14–16
    foreign economic development work of, 13–14
    raw foods discovered by, 9–10
    restaurants/culinary businesses of, 16–18, 137
rutabagas, in rawvioli with mushroom sauce, 97–98

S

SAD (standard American diet), 9, 20, 31–32, 34
salad dressings
    Caesar, 107
    coco-curry sauce, 139–40
    gluten-free house dressing, 114
    Leaf Organics house dressing, 113
    pesto sauce, 137–39
    pomegranate, 116
    for raw slaw, 110
    really raw ranch, 115
    using, 113
salads
    Caesar in the raw, 107–8
    hale kale, 105–6
    holy moly guacamole, 104
    improving, 99–100, 103, 117
    keeping available, 48
    oil use in, 117
    raw slaw, 109–10
    sprouted chickpea hummus, and variations, 100–101
    wakame wonder, 109
    wild rice pilaf, 112
salad spinners, 46
sandwiches
    flying falafel, with coco-curry sauce, 139–40
    See also wraps
sauces
    cheeze, 70–71
    chocolate, 157
    coco-curry, 139–40
    cranberry, 142
    lemon dill, 111
    marinara, 70–71
    mushroom, 97–98
    pesto, 137–38
    raspberry, 149–50
    rawtar, 134–35
    shoyu wasabi, 90
    spicy nut, 132–33
    tahini, 100–101
Schweitzer, Albert, 4
sea veggies, 47
    kelp noodles, 132
    nori rolls with Atlantis pâté, 89–90
    wakame wonder salad, 109
    See also dulse granules
seeds, 47, 54
sesame seeds
    fishless sticks, 134–35
    love loaf, 141–42
    mango bread, 73–74
    Sicilian savory snaps, 65
shish kebab, raw veggie, 136–37
shoyu (nama/raw)
    gluten in, 114
    kreme of mushroom soup, 126
    Leaf Organics house dressing, 113
    Middle Eastern lentil soup, 122
    raw veggie shish kebab marinade, 136–37
    spicy nut sauce, 132–33
    wasabi sauce, 90
Sicilian savory snaps, 65
sides, mashed taters, 143
Simply Raw (film), 35
slaw, raw, 109–10

slicers, spiral, 46
slicing techniques, 49–50
sliders, cashew kreme cheeze, 94
smoothies
    about, 77–78
    coconut mylk for, 79–80
    nut mylk for, 78–79
    as quick food for children, 166–67
    recipes for, 81–82
sodas, 32
soups
    heating, 121
    kreme of asparagus, 125
    kreme of butternut squash, 124
    kreme of mushroom, 126
    Mexican corn chowder, 123
    Middle Eastern lentil, 122
    as quick food for children, 167
    Spanish gazpacho, 127
soy milk, 164
Spanish gazpacho, 127
spices, 47
spinach, in pesto sauce, 137–39
spirulina powder, 80, 84
sprouted chickpea hummus, and variations,
    100–101
Sprouter's Handbook, The (Cairney), 53
sprouts, 6, 23, 45
    chart, 57–59
    equipment for, 53
    health benefits of, 53
    keeping available, 48
    preparation process, 54–56
    as salad booster, 99–100
    seeds for, 54
    yields, 55
    See also specific type
squash, butternut, soup, kreme of, 124
squash, summer
    artisan herb bread, 74–75
    love loaf, 141–42
    pizza pizzazz, 69–71
    potatoless salad with lemon dill sauce, 111
    rawsagna, and variations, 130–31
    raw veggie shish kebab, 136–37

strainers, 46
strawberry/strawberries
    ice kreme, 148
    mousse tartlets, 155–56
    in smoothies, 81–82
strep, 165
stroke, 22
St. Thomas (Virgin Islands), 11–12
sugar, refined, 22, 166
sundae, chocolate brownie, 156–57
sunflower seeds
    coco-curry sauce, 139–40
    fishless sticks, 134–35
    flying falafel croquettes, 66–67
    kreme of butternut squash soup, 124
    love loaf, 141–42
    mango bread, 73–74
    Mediterranean burgers with pesto sauce,
        137–38
    Sicilian savory snaps, 65
    veggie sun burger croquettes, 67–68
sunflower seeds, sprouted
    artisan herb bread, 74–75
    baba ganoush, 95
    bedouin burrito, 118–19
    pizza pizzazz, 69–71
    raw slaw, 110
superfoods, 80
supplements
    DHA, 164, 166
    probiotic, 29
    Vitamin B$_{12}$, 37, 164

T
tahini
    baba ganoush, 95
    flying falafel croquettes, 66–67
    flying falafel sandwich, 139–140
    kreme of butternut squash soup, 124
    Middle Eastern lentil soup, 122
    sauce, 100–101, 139
    sprouted chickpea hummus, 100–101
tartlets, strawberry mousse, 155–56
taters, mashed, 143

tea, 32
Thanksgiving meal, 141–43
There Is a Cure for Diabetes (Cousens), 35
tocotrienol powder, 80, 82
Tolkien, J. R. R., 73
tomatoes
    bedouin burrito, 118–19
    heirloom, with coconut mozzarawla, 92
    marinara sauce, 70–71
    Spanish gazpacho, 127
    wild rice pilaf, 112
tomatoes, sun-dried
    marinara sauce, 70–71
    Mediterranean burgers with pesto sauce,
      137–38
    sprouted chickpea hummus with, 101
transitioning to raw-food diet
    dehydration as useful for, 61
    detoxing/fasting, 42–43
    goal-setting for, 39–40, 43
    overcoming food addictions, 21–22, 40–42
Tree of Life Rejuvenation Center (Patagonia, AZ),
    25, 35–36
tropical granola, 87
tropical trip, 82
Tunisia, 13
turnips, in rawvioli with mushroom sauce, 97–98

U

United Nations Development Program (UNDP),
    13–14

V

vegan diet, 3–4, 37, 164
vegetable gardens, 4–5
vegetarianism, 3–4, 23
veggie shish kebab, raw, 136–37
veggie sun burger croquettes, 67–68
very berry, 82
very berry granola, 86
Virgin Islands, 11–12

virgin piña colada, 82
Vitamin B$_{12}$, 37, 164

W

wakame wonder salad, 109
walnuts
    Atlantis pâté, 89–90
    chocolate brownie sundae, 156–57
    cranberry sauce, 142
    cushy carrot cake, 151–52
    in dessert crusts, 149–50
    Mediterranean burgers with pesto sauce,
      137–38
    rawmesan cheeze, 70–71
    rocky road bananas, 147
wasabi shoyu sauce, 90
water, 33
whipped kreme, 157
Whole Foods Markets, 18
wild rice
    pilaf, 112
    sprouting, 112
willpower, 41
works, the, 82
World Health Organization (WHO), 163–64
wraps
    bedouin burrito, 118–19
    Caesar in the raw, 108
    wild rice pilaf, 112

Y

yams, in love loaf, 141–42
yeast, nutritional
    onion rings, 96
    pizza pizzazz, 70–71
Young, Robert O., 25, 31–32

Z

zucchini
    potatoless salad with lemon dill sauce, 111
    raw veggie shish kebab, 136–37

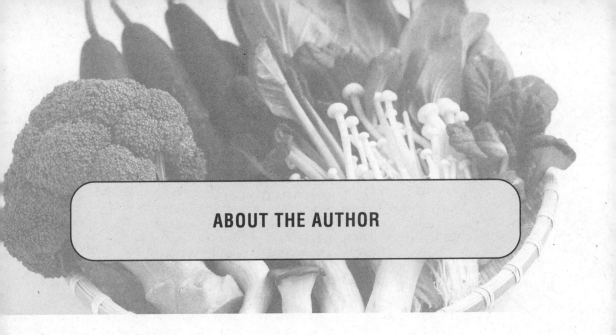

ABOUT THE AUTHOR

A world traveler and culinary eclectic, Rod Rotondi has used his unique experience and perspective to translate world cuisine into delicious and affordable raw, organic, and vegan offerings. Rod's dream was to create an inclusive eatery so affordable and delicious that people would eat there daily and make a positive change to their lives. Thus was born Leaf Organics, one of the first certified-organic restaurants. He owned restaurants in Culver City (from 2004 to 2010) and Sherman Oaks (from 2005 to 2010), both of which received rave reviews. His latest restaurant, Leaf Organics in Los Angeles, serves vegan and raw meals. Rod's catering business offers an array of raw, vegan, and certified-organic entrées, wraps, salads, dips, crackers, and desserts. Rod, who lives in Los Angeles, takes part in many charity events throughout the Los Angeles area hosted by such organizations as Save the Bay, the American Heart Association, and the Breast Cancer Fund. He also speaks at schools and colleges and has catered the Grammy Awards and other entertainment-industry functions. Rod has created *Raw Food for Real People — The DVD*, teaches "uncooking" classes, and is working on a television series. Please see his website at www.leaforganics.com for more information or to buy the DVD, equipment, books, or food items.

NEW WORLD LIBRARY is dedicated to publishing books and other media that inspire and challenge us to improve the quality of our lives and the world.

We are a socially and environmentally aware company, and we strive to embody the ideals presented in our publications. We recognize that we have an ethical responsibility to our customers, our staff members, and our planet.

We serve our customers by creating the finest publications possible on personal growth, creativity, spirituality, wellness, and other areas of emerging importance. We serve New World Library employees with generous benefits, significant profit sharing, and constant encouragement to pursue their most expansive dreams.

As a member of the Green Press Initiative, we print an increasing number of books with soy-based ink on 100 percent postconsumer-waste recycled paper. Also, we power our offices with solar energy and contribute to nonprofit organizations working to make the world a better place for us all.

Our products are available
in bookstores everywhere.
For our catalog, please contact:

New World Library
14 Pamaron Way
Novato, California 94949

Phone: 415-884-2100 or 800-972-6657
Catalog requests: Ext. 50
Orders: Ext. 52
Fax: 415-884-2199
Email: escort@newworldlibrary.com

To subscribe to our electronic newsletter, visit
www.newworldlibrary.com